The Ultimate Vegan Guide

THE ULTIMATE VEGAN GUIDE

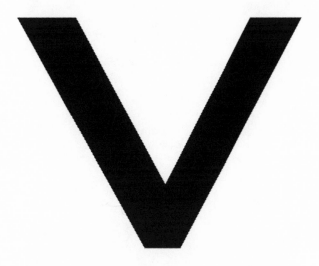

COMPASSIONATE LIVING
WITHOUT SACRIFICE

ERIK MARCUS

Vegan.com • Santa Cruz

Many of the books and food products referenced herein are carried by the Vegan.com grocery. Apart from this association, the author and Vegan.com maintain no financial connection to any product mentioned in this book.

The author and Vegan.com urge you to seek the guidance of a Registered Dietitian or Medical Doctor when making a change of diet. None of the statements in this book are intended to substitute for professional nutritional advice and counseling.

Published by Vegan.com, Santa Cruz, CA.

Printed on acid-free paper in the United States of America.

Cover by John Beske.

Title page, index, and typesetting by the author.

First Edition

For Conrad.
I thought I rescued you,
but it was you who rescued me.

Contents

Acknowledgments

One day, I want to hide myself in a cave for a few months with about ten pounds of coffee, so that I can be the first person to write a nonfiction book that thanks no one. But I find that in the absence of such drastic measures, people inevitably appear in your life who deserve thanks.

My parents, Sonja and David Marcus, always top such a list. They aren't just my parents; they have also served as the foster parents of 300 kittens and counting. Not too many adults have legitimate reason to regard their parents as heroes.

Everyone who visits Vegan.com, or who attends my speaking events, helps me to keep on keeping on. I'm constantly thankful for the friendship and generosity of Paul Kahlon and Sonu Lamba. Tom and Kim Scholz have given my writing and activism every possible sort of support and encouragement.

John Beske created a wonderful cover that I think perfectly captures the spirit of this book. It was an amazing experience to be able to hire a vegan for this critical project and to watch him nail it.

There are a number of dedicated activists whose work on behalf of animals continually inspires me: Nancy Callan, Jodi Chemes, Joe Espinosa, Evelyn Kimber, Michelle Sass, Stewart Solomon, and Dill Ward.

I am lucky to have regular conference calls with Laura Dilley and Michelle Cehn—calls which directly shaped the final chapter and first appendix of this book. Kristen Twombly and her dad Scott closely read a final draft of this book, sending me back to my desk to write a few thousand much-needed words.

I am privileged to frequently communicate with Paul Shapiro, Jack Norris, Matt Ball, Erica Meier, Gil Schwartz, and Nathan Runkle—these amazing people have a real shot at ending factory farming in our lifetimes. Thanks go to David Wolfson for consulting with me on the Common Farming Exemption passage of this book, and for being the first to document this powerful and incredibly sleazy tool of agribusiness.

My old friend Steve Middleton at the Alt. marketing agency offered some helpful thoughts about choosing a book title, and dissuaded me from titling this book: *Principles of Intermediate Accounting, Vol. II.*

Life can end abruptly and without warning, so I'm grateful that I've been granted the time to write this little book.

Introduction

Going vegan can be terrifying, especially at the very beginning when you're wondering what fine mess you've just gotten yourself into. I wrote this book to tell you everything I've learned from twenty years, and counting, as a vegan.

We start with a quick but thorough look at why a vegan diet makes so much sense, and I hope this information increases your motivation to become vegan. Next, we move into the heart of the book: 24 chapters devoted to everything you need to know to be vegan. We then finish off the book by visiting a vital yet neglected part of the vegan lifestyle: activism and outreach.

I hope this book increases your excitement about going vegan, and convinces you that this is a step that you're ready to take.

Part I

Why?

"In what respect, Charlie?"

—Sarah Palin

Chapter 1

Health and the Environment

The practice of avoiding meat dates back thousands of years, but it was not until the mid-1800s that the word vegetarian was coined. Shortly thereafter, people began bickering over who could reasonably call themselves vegetarian. Everyone agreed that vegetarians don't eat the flesh of animals, but beyond this point opinion diverged. One faction advanced the reasonable position that only foods of plant origin—grains, beans, vegetables, fruits, nuts, and so forth—should be called vegetarian. The other side took a less literal approach, and asserted that dairy products and eggs ought to be considered vegetarian as well. When the dairy and egg abstainers objected that this wonderful new word was being wrongfully diluted, they were told to pound sand.

So vegetarianism remained a muddy concept until a hundred years later, when a young Brit named Donald Watson came onto the scene. Realizing that the word vegetarian had become irrevocably associated with milk and eggs, Watson decided to coin a new word. He dropped half the letters from the word vegetarian, thereby creating the word vegan. And this time around, Watson was not going to let those egg and dairy eaters spoil things. He defined vegan to mean a diet that excludes all animal products—meat, fish, dairy products, eggs, and even honey. To promote this new concept, Watson co-founded The Vegan Society in 1944.

The word vegan took decades to catch on, no doubt because it's a singularly dreadful word that manages to annoy and to confuse, especially where pronunciation is concerned. Most people unfamiliar with the word make the reasonable assumption that vegan rhymes with Megan. Others, a minority, decide its G should be soft, and pronounce the word Veh-Jun. Both pronunciations are sensible, but alas, wrong—in coining his word, Donald Watson selected the most counterintuitive pronunciation possible: *Vee-Gen,* with the accent on the first syllable.

If the entire marketing staff at Oscar Mayer had been handed the task of coming up with a geeky and confusing name that would inhibit the spread of plant-based diets, it's hard to imagine them surpassing Watson's effort. Nevertheless, this loathsome and ugly word slowly but surely took hold, and now it's probably too late to get rid of it. But enough about the word vegan—it may be a terrible word, but it's a wonderful concept. Let's now look at why people find this style of eating so worthwhile.

Many people become vegan out of concern for their health or the environment. Let's look at these two subjects in turn.

Health

Speaking broadly, the more animal products a person consumes, the greater the risk of heart disease, diabetes, and certain kinds of cancer. Yet some people can plainly tolerate plenty of meat, milk, and eggs without ultimately paying a price. For others, though, even a comparatively small amount of animal products leads to severe health problems. Based on your family history, you can make an informed guess about where you fall on this spectrum. But in the absence of expensive medical testing, assessing the amount of animal products you can safely eat is still very much a guessing game.

Perhaps the biggest threat posed by animal products is that these foods are a slippery slope where your health is concerned. Nearly all healthy people can likely tolerate a couple roasted pieces of chicken a week without suffering adverse health consequences. The trouble is that it's easy to go from eating a little chicken to making things like ice cream, pepperoni pizza, and burgers a regular part of your diet. Sadly, no alarm bells start ringing when a person passes his or her individual risk threshold. Instead, the damage silently accumulates, year by year, in terms of gradually clogging arteries and significantly increased cancer and diabetes risk.

The beauty of a vegan diet is that it slams the door shut on all animal products, so you never have to wonder if your personal risk threshold has been exceeded. What's more, a well-planned vegan diet eliminates excessive amounts of fat and calories—so it's no surprise that vegans tend to be leaner than the general population, and suffer dramatically lower rates of obesity. And, on top of all this, a vegan diet tends to include far more fruits and vegetables than a typical omnivorous diet. There is a strong correlation between fruit and vegetable consumption and reduced cancer risk.

I don't mean to suggest that the only way to eat healthfully is to become vegan. It's certainly possible to construct an extremely healthful omnivorous diet. But veganism confers unique advantages in terms of keeping some potentially harmful foods out of your diet. If you often find yourself eating too many foods you know aren't healthful, a vegan diet can be just what the doctor ordered. As we'll see in Chapter 5, it's easy to construct a vegan diet that is vastly healthier than the omnivorous diet most Americans eat.

Environment

It's common to hear vegan advocates proclaim that you can't be an environmentalist if you eat meat. Nonsense. Yet this claim does contain a kernel of truth. At issue is the undeniable efficiency of growing food directly for people, instead of cycling it wastefully through farmed animals. The inefficiencies of animal production are two-fold. First, a large portion of animal feed ends up, not as meat or eggs or milk, but as manure. And second, when an animal is killed, well over 30 percent of the carcass weight is inedible—you're stuck with a great deal of blood, bones, skin, and so forth.

The concept of eating lower on the food chain therefore makes enormous environmental sense, and there's no doubt that a vegan diet demands fewer resources to feed an equal number of people. Nowhere is the wastefulness of animal production so extreme as where factory farmed pigs and feedlot cattle are concerned. Here, you're feeding the animals at least five pounds of grain for every pound of meat you get back.

Given that farmed animal production is inherently wasteful, why not make the argument that non-vegetarians are leading the planet to ruin? There are two reasons to treat this topic gingerly. First, it's all in the quantity—that is, it's silly to assert that a person is unleashing massive environmental carnage if they're only eating one cheeseburger every few months. Secondly, animal products vary widely in terms of their impact on the environment. For instance, chickens eat like, well, birds. That is, chickens are vastly more efficient than are pigs or cattle when it comes to converting grain to flesh. And what's more, a high percentage of a chicken's body weight is lean meat, so there's less waste during slaughter and processing.

What's the take-home message? We can conclude with certainty that anyone eating pork or beef on a daily basis is gobbling up a vastly disproportionate share of the planet's resources, and that a switch to a vegan diet would dramatically reduce that person's environmental footprint.

Livestock interests sometimes respond to environmental arguments against their industries by asserting, truthfully enough, that cattle and goats are capable of grazing lands that are too arid, remote, or infertile to be worth farming. Free meat! What could be bad? The trouble with proclaiming the virtues of grazing is that overgrazing quickly becomes a problem, and the effects are devastating. Livestock grazing delivers a raft of negative environmental consequences, displacing wildlife and degrading land. The effects of grazing and overgrazing are an enormously complex subject, and are exhaustively addressed in Lynn Jacobs' tome, *Waste of the West*. To summarize in a single sentence the environmental harm wrought by grazing, in the year 2000 a White House report asserted that: "Improvident grazing... has been the most potent desertification force, in terms of total acreage (351,562 square miles) within the United States."

Just as ranching devastates enormous swaths of the earth, so too does fishing inflict almost immeasurable harm onto the world's oceans. At issue is the fact that the oceans produce surprisingly little fish, when measured against the worldwide appetite of six billion people. In consequence, the vast majority of the world's fisheries are currently in steep decline, with many on the brink of collapse.

The examples of overfishing are heartbreaking. The waters off the coast of Newfoundland were once the greatest cod fishery in the world. But thanks to overfishing, the cod were wiped out. Ever since, that ecosystem seems to have suffered irreversible damage. After more than ten years without commercial fishing in those waters, the cod still have not returned.

While it's true that some fish stocks and varieties are not yet threatened, I think that when the overwhelming and unsustainable exploitation of the world's oceans is taken into account, the sensible response is to choose not to contribute to the problem, and to refrain from eating all seafood.

Vegans must show restraint when talking about environmental issues, and be sure not to push the arguments against animal production further than they deserve to be taken. But where beef and fish are concerned, it's clear that these foods are genuine environmental menaces, deserving almost bottomless scorn.

There's one last issue related to food choices and the environment that merits attention. Meat's connection to global warming has become strong and indisputable. But once again, there are nuances that enter into the picture that necessitate some care when discussing this topic.

The United Nations asserts, probably accurately, that livestock accounts for about 18 percent of all global warming. But it's not right to tar all animal products with the same brush. The principal greenhouse gas produced by farmed animals is methane, and the overwhelming majority of this methane comes from cattle, and, to a lesser extent pigs. Why aren't chickens equally culpable in producing greenhouse gases? We've already seen that chickens are much more efficient than mammals in converting grain to flesh. And better efficiency means that chickens generate comparatively little methane.

It's also worth noting that even though beef and dairy cattle are big contributors to global warming, there are technological fixes on the way. Increasingly, large cattle operations are being outfitted with equipment that extracts methane from manure piles; the gas is then harmlessly burned off and the energy sold to electric utilities. Additionally, there is promising research underway that may one day alter the bacteria in farmed animal intestines so that little or no methane is produced.

Just as we saw in regard to health issues, environmental considerations offer strong but not irrefutable reasons to go vegan. It's certainly possible to be a healthy and environmentally conscious non-vegetarian—if you're willing to do the mental gymnastics that accompany indulging selectively in animal products.

At this point, I know I must be sounding like a wet blanket. Where health and the environment are concerned, the benefits of veganism deserve strong consideration, but an honest presentation of the issues does not offer an overwhelming argument that everyone should abstain from all traces of animal products. There is, however, one argument for being vegan that hits a grand slam home run: the issue of animal cruelty and suffering. We'll look closely at this subject in the following chapter.

Chapter 2

The Ethics of Animal Agribusiness

People become vegan for all sorts of reasons. Some do it out of concern for animals, while others become vegan because of health or environmental considerations. Still others are motivated by spiritual beliefs, or simply out of disgust over the whole idea of eating animal flesh.

I think the best starting point for discussing veganism involves looking at the business side of animal agriculture. By understanding the financial constraints the industry operates under, you'll gain deep insights into exactly what's objectionable about meat, dairy products, and eggs. In my case, I maintain a vegan diet because I'm repulsed by everything animal agribusiness represents. A close look at the industry reveals that it systematically brutalizes billions of animals each year, and then lies to cover up these cruelties. The industry even crafts laws that keep it from being held responsible for its treatment of animals.

The more you look at animal agriculture, the more you'll realize that the practice of raising farmed animals under a commodity system guarantees all manner of unconscionable behavior. What's more, it turns out that the ethical lapses of the egg and dairy industries are at least as profound as those perpetrated by meat producers.

I'm going to spare you the gory details of specific cruelties. Instead, let's simply look at how the business of animal agriculture has evolved over the past fifty years. By understanding the basic economics of animal agriculture, you'll see why widespread acts of cruelty and dishonesty are inevitable. You'll also understand why the industry cannot be trusted to fix these abuses.

Every sector of animal agriculture—beef, chicken, pork, milk, and eggs—has transformed radically since the 1950s. A combination of deliberate government policy and economic forces have practically driven small-scale animal agriculture out of existence. In 1950, it was still quite possible for a small family farm to profitably keep a dozen dairy cows, three or four pigs, and a couple hundred chickens. But those days are long gone—you can't make money raising animals on a small scale anymore, not as a conventional producer anyway. In fact, since 1950 more than 95 percent of chicken producers, pig farmers, and dairies have gone out of business—and the number of remaining animal farms keeps shrinking.

And yet America is producing more meat, milk, and eggs than ever before. That's because today's animal farms can be hundreds of times larger than the small family farms they replaced. The most obvious examples of super-sized farms are in the egg industry. Prior to 1950, most of America's eggs were produced by small flocks of birds raised in coops. It was rare for a farmer to own more than a few thousand hens. Today, there are more than sixty egg companies in the United States that each carry inventories at least one million layer hens.

Likewise, large-scale farming practices have taken over all other sectors of animal agriculture. Modern dairy and pig operations confine hundreds or even thousands of animals on a single piece of property. And cattle feedlots are even bigger; the largest feedlots confine more than 50,000 cattle in one facility. As animal farms have grown larger, they've become increasingly cruel. Today's enormous farms crowd animals to a degree unheard-of in the 1950s. At the same time, agribusiness has discovered ways to eliminate most traditional labor costs. As we're about to see, when fewer people tend more animals, animal suffering increases.

Before we go any further, I want to confront what I call the Big Lie of animal agriculture. Regarding the concerns I've so far raised, animal agriculture consistently offers just one response. And this response sounds so reasonable at first, that it seems to be an honest argument offered in good faith. Repeatedly, animal agriculture asserts that the industry must provide decent care to the animals they raise, and give them comfortable conditions, because sick animals don't grow to their full potential, nor will they be efficient producers of milk or eggs.

As I said, this claim sounds entirely reasonable. But in reality it's worse than untrue—it is a deliberately misleading argument constructed in bad faith. The dishonesty of this argument arises from its implication that there are only two styles of raising animals—either you let them gambol happily on grassy hillsides, or you keep them at the brink of death under conditions comparable to a concentration camp. Obviously, no producer can make money from a shed full of dying animals, so animal producers would have you believe that economic necessity alone guarantees that animals will be raised under comfortable conditions. But a close look at animal agriculture reveals that the opposite is true. Rather than guaranteeing a decent level of care, the economic reality of animal agriculture imposes nonstop misery on nearly every one of America's farmed animals.

Let's look a little more closely at this idea that animals must be treated with decency and care, otherwise they won't grow and produce profitably. Naturally, no animal can survive long if deprived of food, air, or water. But what's remarkable is how terrible farming conditions can be while still delivering acceptably profitable yields and low mortality rates. Indeed, in animal

agriculture, horrifying conditions and profitability are insepara-
bly joined.

The economic reality underlying animal agriculture is that
meat, milk, and eggs are almost pure commodities. And the fact
that these foods are commodities guarantees cruel production
methods. Let's now look more closely at the connection between
commodities and cruelty. Discussion of commodities is admittedly a dreary topic, but a basic understanding about commodities provides us with a window through which we can glimpse
animal agriculture's inherently cruel business structure.

The quickest way to understand commodities is to contrast
them to branded products. Products with strong brand names,
like Coca-Cola or Macintosh computers, typically command a
price premium over generic brands. People happily pay double
the cost of generic sodas to get Coca-Cola, because—rightly or
wrongly—they believe Coke to be a tastier product. Since the
only producer of Coke is the Coca-Cola company, people who
insist on drinking Coke must pay whatever the company charges.
Likewise, Apple can maintain a much fatter profit margin than
other computer companies, since they've convinced millions of
people it's worth paying extra to own a Mac.

In contrast to branded products, commodities are never sold
at hefty markups. Instead, the producers of these goods operate
under razor-thin profit margins. Animal products, even when
sold under a brand name, are still almost pure commodities; indeed pork-bellies are frequently mentioned in economic textbooks
as a classic example of a commodity.

As an example of how commodity pricing has unleashed enormous suffering onto farmed animals, let's look at the egg industry.
Like pork-bellies and every other animal product, eggs are essentially a pure commodity. That is, no matter where a carton of
eggs is produced, each egg looks the same, fries up the same, and
tastes the same.

Now, suppose you are the wholesale buyer working for a supermarket. When it comes to purchasing eggs, your job couldn't be easier. You don't have to worry about which farm produces the nicest looking or tastiest eggs, since as far as consumers are concerned one egg is exactly like another. All you have to do is find the farm that will sell eggs in wholesale quantities at the lowest possible cost.

This one simple fact, that supermarket wholesalers select eggs solely on the basis of price, has shaped the entire egg industry. Farms that can undercut their competitors on price will enjoy almost unlimited demand for their eggs. The remaining egg farms are on borrowed time, since they must either sell their eggs at a loss, or not sell them at all. You can now see why more than 95 percent of egg farms have gone bankrupt over the past half-century, while the surviving egg farms have grown enormous.

The Rise of the Battery Cage

Since the price of unnecessary expenses is bankruptcy, egg producers do everything possible to minimize their costs. So let's now look at the strategies egg producers employ to reduce their production costs. There are two main ways to produce eggs as cheaply as possible: maximize each facility's output, and eliminate unnecessary labor. Maximizing output is an easy trick with an obvious solution—you simply cram as many hens as possible into your building; the more hens go in, the more eggs come out.

In order to house as many hens as possible in each shed, the industry relies on "battery cages." These cages can be stacked up to six high, with each cage stuffed full of birds. A battery cage has approximately the same dimensions as a file cabinet drawer, and egg producers often stock each cage with at least six birds.

After maximizing stocking density, the egg producer must also minimize labor costs. And here, we see the primary appeal of battery cages: these cages allow the producer to do away with nearly all labor requirements.

Traditionally, egg farms required substantial amounts of human labor. The hens had to be fed and given water. Their manure had to be regularly raked up and carted away. And finally, the eggs had to be collected each day. These jobs all demanded a great deal of time. But the introduction of battery cages eliminated all these required tasks at a single stroke.

Battery cages allow the provision of feed and water to be handled mechanically—with the birds all confined in cages, it's a simple matter to bring feed by conveyor belt, and to pipe water to dispensers located in each cage. Likewise, battery cages also eliminate the need to rake away excrement. That's because the bottoms of these cages are constructed of wire rather than sheet metal, and the excrement slips between these wires and falls into the slurry pits dug underneath the sheds.

The most labor-intensive task traditionally done on egg farms involved the daily gathering of eggs. Each day, every hen needed to be lifted up, so that any eggs she was trying to hatch could be taken. It would seem there would be no way to automate the task of gathering eggs, but once again battery cages made human labor obsolete. The wires in the cage flooring, while far enough apart to allow excrement to drop through to the slurry pits, are close enough together that the eggs remain inside the cages. These wire floors are tilted at a slight angle, which means that after an egg is laid, it rolls through a gap at the front of the cage and slips onto a conveyor belt. Once a day the belt is turned on, and the eggs are transported into a room for packing.

From an economic perspective, battery cages are an amazing piece of technology. Cheaply mass-produced, these cages enable egg producers to stock birds at maximum density while simultaneously cutting away nearly all labor costs. There is simply no disputing that battery cages offer the most cost-effective way to produce eggs. But these cost savings come at a staggering price when animal suffering is taken into consideration. In fact, it's hard to conceive of a more inhumane way to house layer hens, or for that matter any animal, than to keep them in battery cages.

If the cruel nature of battery cages isn't evident from the brief description I have provided, one look at any photograph of battery hens will reveal the truth. And that is why, as we'll see later in this chapter, the egg industry works so hard to keep photographs and videos of egg farms from the public eye. For people who see these images or who visit an egg farm in person, the most obvious cruelty relates to the unbelievable degree of crowding that the birds experience. At five or more birds per cage, the floor-space for each bird amounts to less than a single sheet of notebook paper.

Because of this tight confinement, the stressed hens have a tendency to peck at one another. This pecking problem would diminish if the hens were only given more space, but that solution would reduce profits. So instead, egg producers sear off the ends of each hen's beak, so that when pecking occurs serious injury will rarely result—a blunted beak is unlikely to draw blood.

Although intensive crowding is the most visible welfare problem at egg farms, it's far from the greatest cruelty. That distinction goes to an inconspicuous source—the fact that the sides and bottoms of battery cages are constructed of wire. At first glance, the fact that battery cages are constructed of wire seems hardly worthy of mention. But the reality is that from the time a seventeen-week-old hen arrives from the hatchery, she spends every moment of the rest of her life in a battery cage. Her entire adult life is therefore spent either standing on wire or sleeping pressed against it. As the weeks and months pass, the wire eats into her feet, wears away feathers, and digs into her flesh. Most battery hens are kept a minimum of eighteen months in these cages before they are sent to slaughter.

By the time hens have spent a year inside a battery cage, they look like no chicken you would ever imagine. Most of their feathers have been abraded away from the wires. On their bare skin, numerous cuts, scrapes, and sores are plainly visible. Yet the true extent of their suffering and deprivation is only visible when one of these hens is rescued. Standing on soil for the first time, the hen will take loping, unbalanced, tentative steps—after spending nearly all her life inside cramped wire-floored cages, she has forgotten how to walk. She's never seen sunlight, breathed clean air, or pecked in the dirt.

Eggs are among the cheapest foods in America, and without battery cages such low egg prices would be impossible. I believe that no food—not even veal—contains more misery per mouthful than a typical supermarket egg. For each conventionally-produced egg, a hen must spend about thirty hours standing or sleeping on wire.

To say that egg producers have a huge financial incentive to mistreat their animals actually understates the problem. The truth is far worse: under fierce commodity pricing pressure, egg producers *must* either mistreat their animals, or go out of business.

At this point, it's insightful to ask what sort of person would decide to enter an industry that treats animals this way. The answer may be the egg industry's fundamental problem—it attracts emotionally calloused people who have no regard whatsoever for animal suffering. And once ensconced in the industry, competitive pressures force each producer to adopt every cost-cutting step available, no matter how cruel. The economics of the industry mean that there is no room for acts of conscience. To the contrary, the industry is in an ethical race to the bottom—fierce economic pressures guarantee that any producer who takes a stand against cruel production methods will be driven out of business.

Now that we've looked closely at America's egg industry, let's quickly examine the lives of other sorts of farmed animals. We're about to see that the same commodity-driven cost-cutting that has shaped the egg industry generates comparable cruelties where other farmed animals are concerned.

Dairy Cows

The life of a modern dairy cow is one of heartbreaking sadness coupled with constant physical strain. In order for them to produce as much milk as possible, cows are kept pregnant nine months out of every year. And although cows immediately display a strong maternal bond for their young, each newborn calf is forever taken from the mother within just a day or two of birth. There is a small comfort, at least, that the mother cow never learns the fate of her calf: most of the males are either slaughtered immediately, or spend an agonizing few months inside a veal crate. The female calves are commonly raised as dairy cows.

Although the dairy industry popularizes the myth that milk universally comes from happy cows grazing lush hillsides, the reality is that many dairy cows are raised at factory farms. These cows are packed in barren sheds, and are often not allowed outdoors to graze.

Dairy cows never die of old age, they die of middle age. That is, as their milk yields decline with each successive pregnancy, they become unprofitable to keep, and are sent to slaughter.

Beef Cattle

Cattle raised for beef suffer less cruelty than other farmed animals, since they spend at least the first six months of their lives grazing outdoors on the open range. Yet during this time, they suffer branding and de-horning, and the males are castrated. No anesthetic is given for any of this.

As the maturing calves approach adulthood, they are taken from their mothers and trucked to a feedlot. Feedlot conditions are universally appalling. Most facilities are enormous—some contain tens of thousands of cattle. You can often smell a feedlot from miles away, and the ground the animals walk and sleep upon is urine-drenched manure, trampled by thousands of cattle into pitch black filth.

In my previous book *Meat Market*, I wrote: "the business of a feedlot is to trade health for size." This assertion cannot credibly be disputed.

At the feedlot, the cattle are put on all-corn rations and implanted with hormones to speed their growth. This corn-based diet is terribly unhealthy for cattle, and frequently produces liver problems. But there's no doubting that a corn-based diet causes rapid weight gain: at the feedlot, cattle gain almost 100 pounds each month. After four to five months at the feedlot, the bloated animals are trucked to slaughter. The "Meet Your Meat" video, which can be watched online at YouTube, shows the animals' final minutes. I strongly believe that every non-vegetarian has an ethical obligation to watch at least a few minutes of slaughter-house video.

Pigs

In the United States, about half of all pigs are raised in just three states: Iowa, North Carolina, and Minnesota. Agribusiness has taken advantage of weak environmental and anti-cruelty regulations in these states to build massive pig confinement operations.

The unluckiest of all these pigs are the breeder sows, who spend their entire lives in gestation and farrowing crates, pumping out the piglets who will be raised for meat. The crates in which these mother pigs are confined are comparable to veal crates in terms of restricting movement—they are far too narrow to permit a normal range of motion or even to allow the animals to turn around. This extreme confinement is lifelong, and a breeder sow may be kept crated without interruption for several years. The isolation and frustration caused by this unrelenting ordeal frequently results in psychological damage, which is manifested by stereotypies—repetitive, constant, and abnormal movements that are widely accepted by scientists as a sign of profound emotional disturbance.

Unlike their mothers, pigs raised for meat are kept, not in crates, but crowded pens. The packing together of so many young animals into tightly confined areas gives rise to regular conflicts. Specifically, when crowded tightly together, pigs commonly react to this stress by biting at each others' tails. Pig farmers call tail-biting a vice—in effect, blaming the pigs for their response to overcrowding.

The main risk of tail-biting isn't the inevitable nip or bite. It's that pigs in factory farms are so depressed and dispirited that they often won't protest or run away when their tails are bitten. So what pig farmers do to prevent serious tail-biting injuries is amputate each pig's tail, save for a tiny nub. This nub is extraordinarily sensitive, and pigs will go to any length to avoid being bitten. Problem solved, factory farming style: the animals remain crowded and miserable, but lose the capacity to seriously injure one another. Providing the pigs with adequate space would also resolve the tail-biting problem, but this solution is regarded as prohibitively expensive.

Perhaps the most deplorable aspect of pig farms isn't the confinement, but the air quality. Pigs have a far keener sense of smell than humans—more discriminating, in fact, than even dogs. Unfortunately, the stench of concentrated pig manure and urine is one of the most overpowering odors imaginable. The ammonia and dust actually eat into the pigs' lung tissue, and postmortems of slaughtered pigs commonly reveal lesions in the lungs—an especially disturbing fact given that pigs are only about six months old when slaughtered. It's hardly surprising that workers at pig farms are likewise prone to respiratory problems. In fact, the air in and around pig farms is so toxic that even people living nearby these facilities suffer heightened rates of lung disorders.

Meat Chickens

Meat chickens have been specially bred to grow at astonishing speed. These birds grow so quickly that many are slaughtered at just 39 days of age. In otherwise healthy flocks, about 1 to 4 percent of these chickens will die suddenly and prematurely from the bodily stresses brought on by their rapid growth. In the United States alone, we have at least 10 million birds dying suddenly each year because they have deliberately been dealt a defective genetic hand.

The chickens who survive until slaughter spend the six or seven weeks of their lives on a crowded indoor floor. Like pigs, chickens are highly socially-oriented, and they have no problem recognizing each bird in a normal flock of one or two dozen chickens. But this ability, and the social hierarchy that chickens instinctively assemble, breaks down when you've got upwards of 20,000 chickens crowded together in a single shed. It's a noisy, dusty, fear-filled environment where every basic need, apart from eating and drinking, is frustrated.

I once met a chicken who knew his name, and would run to you and jump in your lap when called. And yet agribusiness and the law treat chickens as if they are not sentient beings. When the time comes for slaughter, even the pathetically minimal legal protections extended to cattle and pigs are withheld from chickens. Everything at a chicken slaughterhouse is set up to enable the quickest possible slaughter at the least possible labor cost, with no regard to the suffering this system creates. After the birds are shackled by their feet, most of the remaining processing, including the throat-cutting, is done mechanically. There is no legitimate stunning prior to throat cutting: quite to the contrary, the birds are jolted with electricity so that their heads will momentarily hang limp to permit their throats to be mechanically slashed. Hanging upside down by their feet, while fully conscious, the birds then bleed to death.

Lies and Lawmaking

When you look at how commodity-based pricing dictates conditions at both factory farms and slaughterhouses, the welfare situation for today's farmed animals is easy to analyze. In the United States, what we have is an industry that raises more than ten billion animals each year—run by precisely the people who shouldn't be allowed anywhere near an animal.

In the face of such ubiquitous animal cruelty, what's remarkable is the hostility the industry showers upon any efforts to improve animal welfare. The industry has a two-pronged strategy for dealing with the welfare issue: lie about farmed animal cruelties, and lobby to pass laws that make these cruelties legal.

The distortions and outright lies are in evidence everywhere. California dairy producers have spent millions of dollars on television advertisements depicting beautiful hillside grazing pastures, yet these ads never display the cramped stalls at the state's many dry-lot dairies. Children of my generation even watched Ronald McDonald proclaim during television commercials that the company's hamburgers were actually the fruit of plants growing in "hamburger patches."

But it is the egg industry that deserves the Grand Prize for deceiving consumers about animal welfare. In 2002 America's egg industry decided to tackle the animal welfare issue. The obvious path forward would have been to abolish battery cages, while boosting floor space per bird. This could easily have been done industry-wide, at the behest of the industry's flagship trade group, the United Egg Producers (UEP). About 85 percent of eggs sold in America are produced under UEP guidelines, so a strict set of new welfare standards could have transformed the egg industry overnight.

Instead, the UEP created a snazzy new logo which stated, "Animal Care Certified," with these words encircling a large check mark. Egg producers then proceeded to prominently stamp this logo on just about every carton of eggs sold in the United States. Just one problem remained: the Animal Care Certified program was a sham. It called for a gradual and pathetically insufficient increase in the floor-space per bird, as well as for the phasing out of a cruel practice called forced molting that deliberately deprived birds of food.

But the Animal Care Certified program did nothing to address the egg industry's primary cruelties. Under the program's guidelines, hens would still spend their lives in battery cages, they would still be subjected to beak-searing, and no hen would ever receive individualized veterinary care, no matter how grave the need. In fact, even after the program's phase-in period for expanded cage-space was complete, each hen would still have less cage space than a sheet of notebook paper. In short, the Animal Care Certified program was a gigantic fraud perpetrated against American egg buyers.

Fortunately, the egg industry's deceptive practices did not escape notice. The Better Business Bureau interceded in 2003, and filed a complaint that the Animal Care Certified program was misleading consumers. But since the Bureau lacked authority to shut down the program, the UEP ignored their complaint, and factory farmed eggs continued to be sold using this logo.

But in 2005, the Federal Trade Commission stepped in. Acting on the Better Business Bureau's complaint, the FTC forced the egg industry to abandon its deceptive logo. The industry has since changed their logo's wording to read, "United Egg Producers Certified"—whatever on earth that's supposed to mean.

Beyond deliberately misleading consumers with bogus advertising and public relations campaigns, animal agriculture hires lobbyists to enact laws that perpetuate animal cruelty. Some of these laws are expressly designed to keep activists from documenting conditions at factory farms. Under the guise of fighting terrorism, numerous state laws have recently entered the books that forbid trespassing and photography at factory farms. In fact, in Kansas and Montana, the mere act of bringing a camera into a factory farm or slaughterhouse is a criminal offense.

And while the industry seeks to jail anyone who would dare to document animal cruelty, it also tries to exempt itself from existing animal welfare laws. Its most important effort in this respect has been to get "Common Farming Exemption" (CFE) laws passed in most top agriculture states. Although enacted on the state level, these laws are all written with nearly identical language—suggesting that a highly organized entity with deep pockets has been pulling the strings. Under state CFE laws, it becomes practically impossible to win an animal cruelty case against a factory farm or slaughterhouse. That's because most instances of factory farm cruelty are remarkably widespread—they are cruelties practiced on millions or even billions of animals on an industry-wide basis. These cruelties include: using caustic paste to dehorn dairy cows; castrating pigs and cattle without anesthetic; the beak-searing of chickens; and crowding nearly every type of farmed animal to an unconscionable degree.

And that's where CFE laws work their magic. Under these laws, so long as the cruelty in question is considered "common," "normal," or "customary," within animal agriculture, it is exempt from prosecution. In states that have passed CFE laws, a factory farm can do virtually anything it likes to its animals, as long as other factory farms are behaving similarly. David Wolfson, the animal rights attorney who has extensively documented the existence of CFE laws, says, "Common Farming Exemptions give complete power to the farming community to decide what is cruelty to a farmed animal. If the industry adopts a practice, it automatically becomes legal, and farmers cannot be prosecuted for cruelty, no matter how horrific the practice."

Alternative Animal Agriculture

Much of the cruelty related to factory farmed animal products can be cut away by switching to alternative producers. When more money is put into care, feed, and housing, the welfare of farmed animals can increase markedly. Of course, people who choose this option must pay significantly more for their meat, milk, and eggs.

Unfortunately, much animal suffering simply cannot, under any reasonable circumstances, be removed. Many people become vegan out of distaste for the killing of animals. For people with this motivation, even cage-free eggs and organic milk are unacceptable. Unless they die prematurely of disease, every free-range layer hen, and every organic dairy cow ends up in the slaughterhouse at a young age. That's because milk and eggs are reproductive products, and yields diminish as the animals age. So every drop of organic milk, and every free-range egg sold in stores, comes from an animal who will ultimately have her throat cut.

Slaughter aside, the hour-by-hour misery of farmed animals can indeed be erased, given appropriate care. The trouble is that raising animals humanely demands a great deal of extra money— the better the care, the greater the cost. This in turn gives rise to the problem of accurate labeling. Animal products from alternative producers are uniformly marketed as being humane, as if each of these animals is given the same excellent level of care. Nothing could be further from the truth.

Even outside the factory farm, there remains the constant temptation for producers to cut costs in order to gain a financial edge. And, unfortunately, the existing alternative labels—"free-range," "grass-fed," "organic,"—are so vague in some cases as to be meaningless, especially where animal welfare is concerned. Not only are welfare standards ambiguous, but there is practically no state or federal law enforcement that holds producers responsible for their claims of enhanced welfare. This lack of monitoring opens the door to all manner of abuse. Most consumers are happy to believe that merely by purchasing "free-range" eggs, or "organic" milk, they are doing their part to stamp out animal cruelty. The image these products conjure up are chickens cheerfully pecking the dirt outdoors, and cows munching grass on picturesque hillsides. The reality is often surprisingly bleak.

The trouble is that free-range eggs and organic milk command much higher prices in the market than their factory farmed counterparts. And, tragically, agribusiness is full of ethically challenged people who will do practically anything to an animal to earn an extra dollar. Some of these producers doubtless see the free-range and organic markets as easy money. They can do the bare minimum suggested by these standards, and pocket the extra money these foods command.

How bad does it get? Many "cage-free" and "free-range" layer hens have virtually no opportunity to set foot outdoors. And while the stocking density for these hens generally isn't comparable to what occurs in battery cages, it's still nothing that can fairly be called humane. More abusive still is what occurs at many so-called "organic" dairies. It's true that these cows are given organic feed, and not injected with Bovine Growth Hormone or antibiotics, but many of these organic dairies are nevertheless factory farms by any reasonable definition. At least one of these so-called organic dairies keeps upwards of 6000 cows in cramped stalls, yet still gets away with charging premium prices for their "organic" milk. The lesson here is that so-called "organic" meat, milk, and eggs can still come from factory farms.

Since labeling reveals so little, the onus is on the consumer to determine welfare conditions first-hand. It's time-consuming for consumers to check up on animal welfare standards, since every farm they purchase from needs to be personally investigated— ideally on a regular basis. Plus, the farms that have the best welfare are likely to have higher prices than ersatz "free-range"

and "organic" farms. All of this means that conscientious consumers of animal products must invest considerable time and
money to patronize farms with high welfare standards. When all
this is taken into account, even people who have no problem with
animal slaughter may well decide to chuck it all and just become
vegan. It is *much* easier and cheaper to follow a vegan diet than
it is to perform due diligence on a diet that includes meat, milk,
or eggs.

Even on animal farms with the best welfare, there are still
troubling questions and ugly answers. For instance, what happens to the male counterparts of the female "layer strain" chicks
obtained by a free-range egg farm? Many free-range farms obtain
these females from standard commercial hatcheries. And since
the males in question can neither lay eggs nor economically be
raised for meat, the hatchery may kill them using exceptionally
inhumane methods—the chicks may be smothered in trash bags
or ground up while still alive.

Similarly, what happens to the male offspring of "organic,
pasture fed" dairy cows? All dairy cows are impregnated annually to keep up the flow of milk. The male calves, even those
born at organic farms, are routinely sold at auction to veal farmers. Questions like these can drive a person either to drink, or
to become vegan. But it's precisely because of their unpleasant
and grave implications that these sorts of issues must be personally investigated by every truly conscientious consumer of animal
products.

The Vegan Lifestyle

This chapter offered only a brief look at the enormous industry
of animal agriculture. But the deeper you dig, and the more
you read, the clearer it becomes that factory farming deserves
our disgust and contempt. This industry attracts precisely the
people most unsuited to being entrusted with animals, and then

puts them into a position where they will face financial ruin if they balk at perpetuating cruelty.

As with meat, the production of milk and eggs always entails the slaughter of the animals involved. Additionally, factory-farmed dairy and egg products arguably contain more misery per mouthful than does meat. Some animal suffering—but by no means all of it—can be avoided by choosing animal products that do not come from factory farms. But finding animal products that aren't associated with needless cruelty demands vigilance and money, and it's quite likely easier to simply switch to a vegan diet.

Although this chapter has focused on the connection between economics and animal cruelty, a comparably strong argument for veganism can be made philosophically. That is, there are numerous schools of thought that advance the idea that it's wrong to kill animals—no matter how "humanely"—simply because we like how they taste. Entire books have been devoted to advancing this argument through a variety of philosophical frameworks including utilitarianism, feminism, and moral rights.

Let's finish this look at animal agriculture by considering the big picture. Since most Americans eat more than 2000 chickens and other land animals in their lifetimes, the choice to go vegan eliminates enormous amounts of misery and slaughter. On the other hand, when you take the 10 billion animals slaughtered annually in the United States and subtract 2000, you've still got 10 billion. And that is why following up a vegan diet with a commitment to activism is essential. The final chapter of this book shows how easy and fulfilling it is to take action against animal agriculture. It's my hope that after reading that chapter you'll move beyond merely being vegan to something infinitely more important: becoming an effective and lifelong opponent of animal agriculture.

But the bulk of this book is devoted to bringing you up to speed on everything you need to know to become vegan. You'll learn how to shop for foods, how to outfit your kitchen, what pitfalls to look out for, and so much more. It's quite easy to become vegan, especially if you have someone showing you how to do it. If you're ready to make the switch, I've done everything I can in this book to make becoming vegan as easy, healthful, and fulfilling as possible.

Part II

How?

"As easy as falling down a flight of stairs."

—unknown

Chapter **3**

Crowding, Not Cutting

Every person contemplating a switch to a vegan diet starts by wondering: just how hard is this going to be? Believe it or not, it's all surprisingly easy. And not just easy but fun. If you follow my advice, your diet will become vastly more fulfilling. You'll be eating better, feeling better, and you'll become increasingly excited about having tossed animal products from your life.

I ate meat every day until I was twenty. And not just a little meat, either. I ate meat with every meal, heaping piles of the stuff, plus loads of gooey cheese and eggs. It would be hard to find a more unsuitable candidate for a vegan diet than I once was. But then one day I encountered a video showing cattle in a slaughterhouse. What I witnessed struck me as indefensibly brutal, and I was soon looking for ways to rid meat from my diet.

Later, as I learned about the cruelty in dairy and egg farming, I transitioned to a vegan diet. I know that to the uninitiated, veganism must sound like it takes incredible willpower, but nothing could be further from the truth. I've got to say, the amount of deprivation I feel is zero. That's because my diet as a vegan is so much more diverse and delicious than the way I ate as an omnivore.

Even though it's fun and easy to go vegan, you can still make things needlessly difficult. Here is the most common mistake that new vegans make: they switch to this diet believing that it's all about discipline and cutting things out. They grit their teeth and give up hamburgers, cheese pizzas, yogurt, and a bunch of their favorite foods. And in place of all that, they eat celery sticks.

Well, that's obviously a recipe for disaster. So let me suggest an alternative: don't *cut out* non-veggie foods, *crowd* them out. Your main job throughout this transition will be to sample as many different vegan foods as possible. Will you love each and every one? Of course not. Some foods you'll hate, others you'll like, while still others you'll adore. The more foods you try, the more you'll find to love.

So, for the next few weeks, give yourself every possible advantage and make a point of not letting a single day go by without sampling several new vegan foods. There are all sorts of places where you can discover new vegan foods. Is there a veggie restaurant in your town? Some of these places are so good, and have so many great dishes, you'll feel like you could eat there every day.

Or, perhaps there's a Middle Eastern or Ethiopian restaurant near you. In these cuisines, almost everything that doesn't include meat tends to be vegan. These choices are just the start of your options—See Chapter 15 for many more. If you like to cook, you'll be happy to know that there are all sorts of fantastic vegan cookbooks, which we'll explore in the next chapter of this book.

You can never go wrong by trying out new vegan foods. A month from now, foods that you currently don't even know exist will be some of your very favorites. Consider my story: I'd grown up eating cheeseburgers—I loved them, and I ate them all the time. But one day a friend dragged me to a Middle Eastern place and I had a falafel sandwich on pita bread, and I've never looked back.

Until that day, I had never even heard of falafel, which turned out to be these incredibly great vegan meatballs made out of chickpeas, garlic, and chopped parsley, and fried golden brown. As I ate my first falafel sandwich, I thought: "Wow, this is so much better than a cheeseburger. Why would I ever eat a cheeseburger again when I could eat one of these?"

If you follow my advice, I guarantee that over the next few weeks you'll discover a number of vegan foods that will rock your world, and all the animal products you grew up eating will start getting crowded out of your diet. Going vegan is not about deprivation, it's about discovery! So keep reading and let me teach you the most important things I've learned about switching to a vegan diet.

Chapter **4**

Cookbooks

After reading the previous chapter, I hope you've committed yourself to trying as many new vegan foods as possible. One of the best ways to sample a constant stream of new foods is to get busy in the kitchen trying out new recipes. But all recipes are not created equal, so this chapter will be about helping you find the ones most worthy of your time.

I have good reason for bringing up this subject so early in this book. The sooner I can turn you on to some great sources of recipes, the quicker you'll gain confidence that switching to a vegan diet is not a big deal. So, the question is, how do you find tasty vegan recipes that won't force you to spend all afternoon slaving away in the kitchen?

Maybe the best place to start is with the Top 10 Recipes collection that I've published at Vegan.com[1] , since these recipes are free and are hand-picked favorites from some of the best cookbook authors publishing today. After checking out these recipes, you might be tempted to get all your recipes online. After all, there are seemingly millions of recipes available for free on the Internet. A quick Internet search using the keywords *vegan recipes*

---

[1]http://www.vegan.com/recipes/

will return enough such recipes to keep you busy in the kitchen for decades.

As tempting as it may be to get all your recipes for free, I urge you not to waste time trying random recipes you've found online. Instead, you'll be much better off spending ten or twenty dollars on a great vegan cookbook.

But isn't it throwing money away to pay for a cookbook when the Internet offers thousands and thousands of vegan recipes for free? Well, let's step back and think for a minute about the nature of Internet publishing. Perhaps the most amazing thing about the Web is that anyone, at essentially no cost, can publish anything online for all the world to see. And just as anyone can publish *anything* online, the Internet allows for the publication of *any recipe*, no matter how great or how dreadful. And is a free recipe really a bargain if you've invested five or ten dollars in food, spent an hour or two in the kitchen, and at the end of it your meal doesn't turn out right? No, if you're going to take the time and expense to cook something, it's insane to use a recipe you can't count on to produce terrific results.

There are undoubtedly some fantastic recipes online, but it's often impossible to pick them out from the slew of second-rate offerings.

So what I suggest is that you cook exclusively from vegan cookbooks. With that said, I've got yet another word of warning: there are plenty of mediocre vegan cookbooks out there. I've seen vegan cookbooks with recipes that violate even the most elementary cooking principles.

The problem here is that very few cookbook publishers take the trouble and expense to test every recipe in a cookbook before publication. Fortunately, though, professionalism does exist within the cookbook industry, you just have to find authors who care enough to obsessively test their recipes until they're perfect. Those authors are out there. They include folks like Robin Robertson, Nava Atlas, Mark Reinfeld, Jennifer Raymond, and

Dreena Burton. Buy any cookbook from any of these people, open to a random page, and you can be certain the recipe will turn out just right.

So let me suggest what I consider the perfect first vegan cookbook to buy: *The Quick-Fix Vegetarian* by Robin Robertson. Every recipe in this cookbook is simple and straightforward, and most take just a half-hour or less to prepare.

It's common for new vegans to think they need a shelf-full of cookbooks, but this one book is really all you need to get going. For a measly $12 through Amazon.com, you get 150 delicious, super easy, and healthful vegan recipes. Get this one book and you're done.

Suppose you have a little extra money to spend, and want a more extensive recipe collection. In that case, I'd recommend another book by Robin Robertson, titled *Vegan Planet*. The recipes here are still simple, but they're slightly more involved than those published in her Quick-Fix book. *Vegan Planet* is by far the best value in the vegan cookbook world. At fifteen dollars (again, after Amazon.com's discount), you get a book nearly as thick as a big-city phone directory: 600 pages of recipes, each one guaranteed to turn out just right.

One final recommendation: I'm deeply impressed by a recent cookbook, edited by Linda Long, titled, *Great Chefs Cook Vegan*. What Long has done is solicit 25 of the world's most famous chefs for their favorite vegan recipes. It's a spectacular collection, with every single recipe created by someone who *really* knows how to cook. The recipes tend to be fancier and tougher than what's in either of the Robertson books, and aren't really suited for everyday cooking. But when you want to prepare something super special, these recipes are well worth the time.

The people who succeed at going vegan are the people who give themselves every possible advantage. The sooner you get your hands on a quality vegan cookbook that emphasizes simple recipes, the sooner you'll benefit from a ton of new cooking ideas.

I find it immensely worthwhile to leaf through a great vegan cookbook, even if I have no intention of making any of the recipes. It gets the wheels turning and, in no time at all, I have ideas for a whole bunch of meals I want to try. And remember, every time you discover a new vegan food you love, you're another big step closer to becoming vegan.

Chapter 5

Vegan Nutrition

Switching to a vegan diet can deliver some real health benefits. Compared to a typical omnivorous diet, a vegan diet is generally lower in fat, especially saturated fat. Vegans also usually eat more health-promoting fruits and veggies than omnivores, and they don't have to worry about the scary carcinogens that may form when meat is cooked.

Many vegans therefore have a cavalier attitude about nutrition, reasoning that they eat a far healthier variety of foods than they did as omnivores. While this may in fact be true, it's nevertheless quite possible to develop a variety of nutrient deficiencies on a vegan diet. What's worse, some of these deficiencies can creep up on you—they may take years to manifest, and by the time you realize something's wrong, irreversible damage may have occurred.

This is not a comprehensive book on vegan nutrition, and I have no credentials concerning the subject. My intention in writing this chapter is to tell you some of the most important things to watch out for, and to direct you to some reliable sources of information about nutrition. It's indeed the case that anyone who puts some time into studying vegan nutrition can construct a diet that is vastly healthier than what the typical omnivore eats. The first step to understanding vegan nutrition is to learn which nutrients merit special attention.

So let's look at the main deficiencies that can develop on a vegan diet:

- **Vitamin B_{12}.** The 800 pound gorilla of potential nutrient deficiencies for vegans. There is essentially no B_{12} present in any vegan food, so supplements or B_{12} fortified foods are absolutely necessary. The scariest thing about B_{12} deficiencies is that they can take years to develop. But once symptoms of a B_{12} deficiency appear, the effects can be devastating and can even involve permanent nerve or neurological damage. Believe me, this is one nutrient you need to take seriously, and you need to make sure you take it every day. Luckily, there are a number of vegan B_{12} supplements, and some foods are also fortified with substantial amounts of B_{12}. You'll occasionally run into people who will assert that you can get B_{12} from unfortified vegan foods; ignore these people at all costs.

- **Calories and Protein.** If you eat a lot of low-calorie foods, like fruits and vegetables, you might have trouble getting adequate calories. And while its rare for vegans to get insufficient protein, this can occur on certain diets, especially those that are very low in calories. Some protein-rich vegan foods are: beans, peas, nuts, tofu, and tempeh.

- **Iron.** Many vegan foods, including leafy greens and certain kinds of beans, are abundant in iron. However, menstruating women may have trouble obtaining adequate iron through food alone, and may need to take a supplement.

- **Omega 3s and DHA.** Since fish provide most of the Omega 3s in a typical omnivorous diet, vegetarians and vegans need to seek out other sources of this nutrient. Omega 3 needs can be satisfied by eating ground flax seeds stirred into smoothies or soymilk, or by making salad dressings that contain flax oil. Note that flax seeds must be ground before they are eaten; otherwise their Omega 3s won't be absorbed. Also, flax oil must be kept refrigerated and should never be heated, since it breaks down during cooking. Since flax oil goes rancid quickly, don't buy more than a few weeks' worth of oil at a time, and always keep it refrigerated. You should take 1-2 tablespoons of ground flax, or 1-2 teaspoons of flax oil daily. Finally, since some people don't naturally convert enough of their Omega 3s into DHA, it can be wise to also regularly take a vegan DHA capsule.

- **Vitamin D.** Many Americans don't get enough Vitamin D, and since most Westerners get much of their Vitamin D from fortified milk, vegans can develop a deficiency here unless they find a reliable source. This might include fortified soymilk or a multivitamin. You should be aiming to consume 25 micrograms of Vitamin D every day. If you get a lot of exposure to direct sunlight, you can also meet your Vitamin D needs that way—but be wary of overdoing sun exposure, since it can prematurely age skin and lead to skin cancer.

- **Iodine.** An essential nutrient that can be in short supply in a vegan diet. Courting an iodine deficiency is not something you want to mess with unless the idea of a large goiter forming on your neck sounds appealing. Most Westerners get their iodine either from iodized salt or from milk—it's pretty scarce in other foods, with the exception of seaweed. So if you follow a vegan diet containing non-iodized salt and no sea vegetables, you can easily get into trouble. It's wise to take a daily multivitamin containing iodine, and to boost your intake by eating some form of seaweed at least a few times a month.

- **Calcium.** A poorly-planned vegan diet may provide insufficient calcium. Fortunately, many green leafy vegetables are loaded with calcium, as is broccoli. Calcium-fortified orange juice and soymilk are two more great sources of this nutrient. Vegan calcium supplements are a valuable option if you are unable to meet your calcium needs through food.

- **Zinc.** It's sensible to take a daily multivitamin that contains zinc, since obtaining adequate amounts of this mineral from vegan foods can be difficult.

I hope the material I've presented in this chapter has persuaded you that nutrient deficiencies can happen to anyone, even vegans. So if you're going to be vegan, it's well worth your time to spend at least an hour or two reading about nutrition. In a relatively short amount of time, you'll learn enough to optimize your diet—and to cut out the risks of developing a deficiency. Isn't it worth a little reading to make sure your diet is the best it can be?

So where do you go to learn more about vegan nutrition? The best single source I've found is the VeganHealth.org website, which is run by Jack Norris. Jack's a registered dietitian who focuses his practice on studying the nutrient deficiencies vegans may be prone to, and he offers comprehensive advice on how to avoid these deficiencies. His website has a couple dozen heavily footnoted articles covering every nutrient of concern to vegans. One of the best things you can do for yourself is to bookmark VeganHealth.org and make a point of reading every article there. Doing so might take you fifteen minutes a day for a couple of weeks, but the things you'll learn from this small effort will benefit you for a lifetime.

If you want to read a book on vegan nutrition, *Becoming Vegan* by Davis and Melina is by far the most popular title, and it's a worthwhile read. If you read Jack's site plus *Becoming Vegan*, you'll know more about nutrition than 99 percent of Americans, and you'll be able to construct a diet that's amazingly healthy.

As we've seen in this short chapter, a bit of time spent reading up on nutrition can pay big dividends. This is one occasion where ignorance is not bliss—why put yourself needlessly at risk of developing a nutrient deficiency? Even if you don't care about your health, it's worth eating right for the animals: there's nothing that dairy industry flacks love more than to publicize occurrences of vegans who develop nutrient deficiencies.

Finally, keep in mind that nutritional needs are especially important during pregnancy, infancy, and childhood. And, at these times, following a vegan diet may pose unique challenges. It's therefore vital for couples wanting to have children to read up on vegan nutrition, and to make sure their children receive every possible advantage from the moment they are conceived.

Chapter **6**

Eat More Produce

The previous chapter looked at the negative side of a vegan diet—we confronted the main nutritional pitfalls and considered ways to minimize your risk of developing a deficiency. Now let's look at the positive side of things: the simple steps you can take to make your diet as healthful as possible.

It's hard to say which the greater health advantage of veganism is: whether it's the fact that on a vegan diet you're not exposing yourself to fatty meats, potential carcinogens, and substantial amounts of saturated fat—or whether the greatest health advantage is that you'll tend to eat a lot more health-promoting fruits and vegetables.

If there's one thing that nutrition researchers are absolutely sure of, it's that people who eat more fruits and vegetables enjoy better overall health, and have lower rates of cancer. Sadly, studies continually show that Westerners eat far fewer fruits and vegetables than they should.

The wonderful thing about becoming vegan is that it gives you an unequalled opportunity to upgrade your diet in various ways. Since you've got to eat something in place of the meat, dairy products, and eggs you formerly ate, why not make a point of stepping up your consumption of fruits and veggies?

One great way to improve your diet is to set goals. If you're not in the habit of eating much produce, why not set a goal to eat ten different kinds of fruits and veggies this week? A goal like this probably sounds impossible to some people, but in reality it's incredibly easy. Just visit your local market, and buy an apple, a pear, some grapes, a tangerine, and a tomato—and boom, you're halfway there. If summer fruit is in season, load up on that as well. The point is to get into the habit of eating several different fruits and veggies every day.

Let me give you another tip that can dramatically improve your overall diet. Many Americans, even those who love veg-etables, are scared off by leafy greens. In a way, that's under-standable. In their raw form, some leafy greens look downright intimidating. Raw kale, for instance, doesn't look like people food, it looks like something you would feed to a goat.

But in reality, there's almost nothing easier to prepare or more delicious than leafy greens. Cut them up, stir-fry the coarsely-sliced stem portions in some olive oil for a few minutes, add in the leafy parts for another minute or two, then quickly sauté some minced ginger and garlic, squirt in a little tamari and you're in business. The whole effort might take you ten min-utes. I personally try to eat a big serving of stir-fried leafy green vegetables every day.

A quick note about spinach. Spinach is usually grown in very sandy soil and often has a beach's worth of sand sticking to its leaves and stems. It therefore needs to be washed thoroughly and repeatedly. And, in contrast to other leafy greens, spinach cooks in seconds rather than minutes. I always discard the stems of spinach when stir-frying.

I've got one other way I love to prepare green leafies: I stir-fry them as I've already mentioned, skip the garlic, ginger, and tamari, and instead mix in some Annie's Goddess Dressing imme-diately before serving. I generally detest bottled salad dressings, but this Annie's Goddess Dressing product goes wonderfully with greens, and you can buy it in any natural food store or from Amazon.com. Just be sure to get the regular Goddess dressing, since other varieties of Goddess dressing may not be vegan.

To conclude this chapter, let me take you through the main leafy greens you can get at any market. There's red, green, or gold chard, collard greens, spinach, mustard greens, and several varieties of kale—from red to green to dinosaur. I go out of my way to eat as much kale as possible, since it's high in both iron and calcium and it's also low in oxalates, which inhibit calcium absorption.

The very best place to buy your leafy greens, and most of your other produce for that matter, is at your local farmer's market. I've devoted Chapter 13 of this book to telling you all about farmers' markets.

Leafy green vegetables are super low in calories and they digest quickly—you may therefore want to serve them over brown rice so the meal will stick to your ribs. Here's a final suggestion: go to your local market or your farmer's market and buy four or five bunches of leafy greens, and make a point of using them all up over the course of a week. As I said, they're delicious and about the healthiest thing you can eat. And once you get into the habit of eating leafy greens every day, you'll have taken another big step towards eating a supremely healthful vegan diet.

Chapter 7

Should vs. Must

We have already covered a lot of ground. We've seen, for instance, that all vegans need a daily source of Vitamin B_{12} and Omega 3s, and that it's a good idea for many vegans to take a multivitamin to guard against other deficiencies, particularly Vitamin D, iodine, zinc, and perhaps iron. We've also seen the benefits of eating plenty of fruits and vegetables every day.

From all this, perhaps you're thinking something like, "It would be a good idea for me to start taking flax for my Omega 3s, and I'll see if I can find some B_{12} somewhere. I really should make a point of taking this stuff."

Well, I don't know if the road to hell is really paved with good intentions, but the road to an inadequate diet certainly is. So before we move on to other subjects, I want to emphasize as strongly as I can that proper nutrition is *not* optional.

In one of his books, Anthony Robbins presents a simple idea that has changed my life: he makes a strong distinction between the word "should" and the word "must." There are all sorts of things in your life and mine that we tell ourselves we *should* be doing, but that we never get around to completing. But when you elevate something to a *must*, you become unwilling to flake out. For instance, you and I probably share at least one must.

Before leaving the house in the morning, we simply must brush our teeth. It doesn't matter if we're tired, or running late, or feeling annoyed, or whatever. We've decided that the importance of brushing our teeth before leaving the house in the morning outweighs any priority other than escaping the house if it's on fire.

So don't let a wimpy word like "should" be all that's in place to ensure that you receive adequate nutrition. It's silly to risk your health, when the commitment to guarantee proper nutrition amounts to just a couple minutes a day. If you're going to make the effort to be vegan, isn't it worth resolving that, every day and without fail, you're going to take in the nutrients your body needs?

With that in mind, let me tell you a few things I do every day to ensure my nutritional needs are covered. I like to use my morning rituals to get my difficult-to-obtain nutrients out of the way. So every morning when I wake up, I make sure to get my Omega 3's. If you're poor, the easiest way to do this is to grind up a couple tablespoons of flax seeds in a $10 propeller-style coffee grinder and stir them into your soymilk. I also take a multivitamin with zinc; mine doesn't have iron since I eat plenty of leafy greens and have never had any indication of being anemic, but if I were a woman of childbearing age I might take a multivitamin with iron. And, finally, I let a sublingual B_{12} tablet sit under my tongue a couple times a week.

If you have the extra money to spend, you should consider taking a vegan DHA supplement in addition to your flax, since some people have trouble converting their Omega 3s into DHA. Also, if you haven't eaten fish for months or years, and you haven't been taking in any flax, there's evidence to suggest you would benefit by taking DHA for at least a few months, in addition to your flax. Amazon.com sells a vegan DHA product made by Deva Vegan Vitamins that costs only $10 a month.

These are all personal musts for me. And I hope you'll consider these steps musts as well. The vitamins and flax seeds I consume cost only about $5 a month, and even if you add in a vegan DHA supplement taken daily, you still come in at about $15 a month. Considering how far these steps will take you in protecting your health, the cost is absolutely trivial.

Now, in addition to my musts, let me share a couple of habits that further improve my overall nutrition. I'm a big fan of eating some fruit first thing in the morning: an apple, a banana, an orange, whatever. When I'm done eating this fruit, I'll have a small handful of nuts.

So before I've even started my day, I've already consumed a significant amount of healthful produce. And since a small amount of nuts eaten daily is associated with better health, I've gotten that out of the way too.

And finally, as long as I'm not driving anywhere, I try to have a glass of wine or beer, and only a glass, with dinner each night. There are countless studies that indicate that a small amount of alcohol taken daily substantially reduces the risk of heart attacks. In fact, a serving of alcohol every day delivers benefits comparable to taking statins, for less money and at lower risk to health. You might think twice about drinking daily, though, if you've got alchoholism in your family—I couldn't bear the thought of prodding anyone predisposed to alcoholism down that awful road.

Since I have a nasty family history on both sides where heart disease is concerned, I try to make it a habit of drinking that daily glass of booze. Hopefully a vegan diet will do much to reduce my chance of heart problems, and it could well be that a small amount of alcohol will put me over the top in overcoming my risk.

Once in a while I'll forget my daily drink, since it's not quite a must as far as I'm concerned. But the vitamin and flax regimen I've talked about here is a must, each day and every day. And it should be for you, too.

Chapter **8**

The Mental Game

Let's now turn to the mental games that everyone plays when moving towards a vegan diet. Becoming vegan obviously involves changing what you eat, but that's only half the challenge. The other half is the mental component: cultivating thoughts and strategies that will make you increasingly confident and happy about embracing a vegan lifestyle.

We live in a meat-based culture, and so it's only natural to pick up ideas and beliefs during your lifetime that will complicate the task of becoming vegan. Happily, there are strategies you can adopt that will overcome your mental obstacles.

Let's start by addressing your fears head-on, and defining your current limitations in the most productive possible way.

Acknowledging Your Fears

Chances are you have some concerns about what life as a vegan would be like. You might be able to precisely identify your fears, or perhaps you just have a vague sense of dread. Whatever the case, I invite you to stop reading now and ask yourself this helpful question: what specific fears do you have about becoming vegan?

Now would be a great time to write down your vegan-related fears on a scrap of paper, and use it as a bookmark while reading this book. Here are some of the most common fears that people have about becoming vegan:

- I will end up going hungry at social gatherings.

- My health could suffer.

- I won't eat well when I travel.

- My spouse won't be supportive.

Whatever your fears, try to articulate them as specifically as possible. Since this book covers all aspects of becoming vegan, any fears you currently have will likely be addressed in the pages that follow. So putting your fears in writing now will provide a big dose of encouragement later on, when you have a chance to compare your initial fears to the things that you've learned from this book.

Most people who have decided to become vegan feel some anxiety about making the change. And that's totally understandable. After all, becoming vegan typically requires jettisoning many of the foods you grew up with, and putting a whole bunch of unfamiliar foods in their place.

It's OK to feel some anxiety at first—in fact, it would be strange if you weren't at least a little nervous. So to start out, let's compare becoming vegan to some things you have already accomplished. I want you to think of some skill that you learned recently or long ago—perhaps riding a bicycle, hitting a baseball, or learning to knit. These are all skills that anyone can learn given a little time and attention. Becoming vegan is very similar. Like taking up yoga or playing guitar, successful vegan eating is basically a learned skill. And, compared to other skills you've doubtless already mastered, switching to a satisfying vegan diet is surprisingly easy. With the effort required to become an atrocious guitar player, you could instead gracefully and healthfully transition to a vegan diet.

It's interesting to hear non-vegans speculate about what life as a vegan must be like. Very often, you'll hear them use the tiniest of issues put forward as a blanket statement about why a person could never become vegan. Let's look at how people articulate their limitations in ways that make a vegan lifestyle appear far harder than it actually is.

Narrowly Define Your Limits

Assuming you're not ready to switch to a 100 percent vegan diet overnight, it makes sense to figure out the areas that are holding you back. I suggest you spend a couple minutes right now thinking about the main obstacles you have.

The reason I recommend that you spend time thinking about your limits is because, by doing so, you can avoid a couple of traps that people fall into. The first trap has to do with language. A lot of people use words like "can't," or worse, "I could never" when it comes to taking steps toward a vegan diet. Language like that is terribly counterproductive. A better way to phrase matters is to use the words, "I'm not yet ready to..."

Please put this book down for a few minutes and write up your list of "I'm not yet ready to..." items.

Once you've got this list in hand, I want to help you avoid the other big trap that people fall into regarding how they set their limitations. In many cases, people set their limitations far too broadly. I was once guilty of doing this too, so I want to show you how I dealt with one of my limits.

When I first started thinking about going vegan, I knew that giving up dairy products was going to be my most significant challenge. I had grown up eating these foods with practically every meal, and so I couldn't dream of going dairy-free overnight. My initial thoughts concerning quitting milk and dairy products could be phrased like this:

I'm not yet ready to give up dairy products.

It's hard to travel far down the vegan path with such a broadly worded limitation. So I had to ask myself: did I like all dairy products equally? On any given day, I might drink milk, eat ice cream, or have cheese on a sandwich. How did I feel about these foods?

The truth was I never liked the taste of milk. On the other hand, I was fond of ice cream but hardly ever craved it. So parting with milk would be easy, while ice cream would be a bit tougher but still do-able. But cheese was another thing entirely. I adored cheese. Realizing this, it made sense to reword my limitation as:

I'm not yet ready to give up cheese.

Now, I was making headway! What a difference between being unready to give up all dairy products, and being unready to give up cheese. But could I go even further? I next asked myself: "Well, do I love all cheese equally?"

Once again, the answer was simple: absolutely not. I loved mozzarella cheese on pizzas. Swiss cheese was OK on sandwiches. Kraft American cheese slices sucked. And Brie was just too revolting for me to contemplate eating. I decided that I could cheerfully give up all cheese except when I ate pizza.

With that decision, I was again ready to further refine my limitation:

I'm not yet ready to give up cheese pizzas.

You can already see what a long way I'd gone from being unready to give up dairy products, to being merely unready to give up cheese pizzas. But I wasn't done yet. I thought about the cheese pizzas I could get locally (I was living in Santa Cruz, California.) In my town, I could get Round Table pizza, which was very good. I could get pizza from Domino's, which was mediocre. Or, I could visit Pizza-My-Heart, which was a locally-owned pizzeria that baked the best pies I'd ever eaten. I decided that I could happily give up Domino's and Round Table pizza if I could still be allowed to eat the occasional slice of cheese pizza at Pizza-My-Heart. So my limitation was once again narrowed:

> *I am not yet ready to give up cheese pizza from Pizza-My-Heart.*

As the months went by, having that occasional slice of cheese pizza seemed less and less special. I was discovering all sorts of vegan foods that tasted every bit as wonderful as the cheese pizzas at Pizza-My-Heart. In short order, I decided I no longer wanted to eat cheese pizza—and this decision was so effortless as to be anticlimactic.

Thanks to my setting clear and narrowly defined limits during my transition to a vegan diet, dairy products did not conquer me; I conquered dairy products.

***

I hope my pizza story shows how helpful it is to put your limitations in writing, and to spend time getting them as clear and narrow as possible.

In your effort to become vegan, you may find that you have limits related to specific foods, to travel, or to social situations. The broader and fuzzier your limitations, the more difficulties you'll face in going vegan. It really doesn't matter how many limits you have at first: by working through the process of defining each limitation in the narrowest possible terms, you'll be preventing these limits from needlessly impeding your progress. Just by doing this simple exercise, you'll likely take several giant steps toward becoming vegan.

Making New Commitments

One happy consequence of narrowly defining what you're *not* ready for, is that this process puts you in a position to recognize the commitments you *are* ready to make. You might be at the point where you're able to contemplate making commitments like these:

- I'm ready to give up eggs.

- I'm ready to give up all dairy products except for cream in my coffee.

- I'm ready to purchase only non-leather shoes.

Let's end this chapter with one final possible commitment that I personally found enormously helpful. During my junior year of college, I was vegetarian but not yet vegan. I didn't feel ready to be all vegan, all the time. But I had just moved into a new house, and I decided that I was ready to be vegan at home. What this commitment accomplished is that suddenly all the groceries I brought into my house became vegan. My vegan cooking skills therefore began improving by leaps and bounds.

This in turn led to me trying more and more vegan foods, and to become ever more comfortable being vegan 90 percent of the time. Within just a few months, I realized I could be vegan outside my house with no special effort. And with that insight, my transition to being vegan was complete.

Chapter **9**

Celebrating Your Progress

As you continue to put effort towards being vegan, it's wise to periodically pause and evaluate the progress you've made. Pausing occasionally to reflect on your progress will not only provide encouragement about how far you've come, it will also enable you to decide what you're ready to do next. I recommend that you periodically ask yourself questions like these:

- What fruits and vegetables did I recently eat that weren't a regular part of my diet in the past?

- What vegan foods have I discovered lately that I especially enjoy?

- What cookbooks and kitchen items have I purchased that will help me create delicious new foods?

- What vegan-friendly restaurants have I dined at recently?

Asking yourself these sorts of questions will help you to recognize the little victories you've achieved. The key to maintaining your enthusiasm during your transition to a vegan diet is to continually recognize, and celebrate, the progress you're making.

Some of your victories are easy to miss, but are well worth noting. Perhaps you ordered some vegan multivitamins or sublingual Vitamin B_{12} tablets? Or maybe you've recently bought some flax seeds and a coffee grinder, or some vegan DHA capsules? If so, you've already taken steps to safeguard your health over the long term, and that's worthy of celebration.

If, after reflecting on your recent efforts, you feel like you've made little progress, don't beat yourself up. Just resolve that this upcoming week will be different. You'll take care of getting your vitamin and Omega 3 situation resolved. You'll get ahold of a great vegan cookbook full of easy recipes. And you'll go out of your way to try a bunch of vegan foods over the next several days, so that the next time you take stock of your progress you'll have ample reason to celebrate.

One of most surprising things about becoming vegan is that you can accurately measure your progress from one week to the next. And what's more, you can resolve to pick up the pace anytime you wish. You can, for instance, decide to try more foods this week than last week. If you've already purchased a vegan cookbook, why not put it on your pillow right now and resolve to browse through it before bed? If there's a veggie-friendly restaurant in your town, how about scheduling a dinner there sometime this week? If you're not yet eating much in the way of fruits and vegetables, you can decide right now to include more fresh produce in your diet.

I hope you're starting to see the value of setting aside ten minutes a week for taking stock of your progress and making new commitments. Whether you accomplished a little or a lot lately, you can decide anytime to take things up several notches for the coming week. Imagine how you'll feel a week from now, when you pause and reflect on your progress, and recognize the great strides you've made.

Things get progressively easier as you discover new foods and learn more about being vegan. I know that at first it may be hard to believe, but you will ultimately reach the point where being vegan becomes second nature. At that point, being vegan involves no extra effort, no feelings of sacrifice, and not even any conscious thought. Whenever you're hungry, the first food that pops into your mind will be healthy, delicious, and vegan.

Chapter 10

The Counterculture

We've spent the last few chapters looking at some of the main issues surrounding the switch to a vegan diet. Now let's look at the bigger picture. In this chapter, we will see how a simple concept pioneered by the counterculture can guide and improve your food choices. You see, almost every Westerner who eats a veggie diet owes a debt to the Vietnam war era counterculture. Oddly enough, it was America's 1960s and 1970s counterculture that produced one of the best ideas guiding the spread of vegetarian eating.

If there was one defining sentiment among young people during that era, it was a distrust for any sort of authority, regardless of whether that authority came from the military, business, school, or the police. There were two main reasons for this distrust: the Vietnam war and the rise of psychedelics.

Vietnam led to sustained outrage from the American public. Any young American man who wasn't politically well connected, or didn't flee to Canada, was likely to be drafted. And over the course of the war, nearly 60,000 American troops died. The American public, particularly the young, was also disgusted by the atrocities inflicted on the Vietnamese, which ranged from civilian massacres to setting entire villages ablaze with napalm.

There's nothing like an unpopular war to fuel rampant public distrust of authority. At the same time, the spread of LSD in America's youth culture added fuel to the fire. If there's one thing that LSD can be counted on to accomplish, it's to undermine the belief that the socially sanctioned way of seeing the world is based on an objective reality.

Between the antiwar movement and the psychedelic drug culture, by the 1970s a substantial percentage of America's youth had adopted a set of values fundamentally at odds with that of their parents' generation. These values embraced pacifism, drug use, sexual permissiveness, and the emergence of a strong protest culture. The glue that held all of this together was a distrust of authority, and along with that came a deep-seated hostility toward everything having to do with capitalism and business. At the time, one of the most cutting insults you could dish out was to suggest that a young person cared about money.

If there was a single term that came to embody the split between the establishment and the counterculture, it was the phrase, "The Man." The Man was shorthand for every sort of business, government, police, or authority figure—anybody who made a profit from and had a vested interest in maintaining the existing order of things.

As the Vietnam war continued to grind away, and all efforts to stop it failed, the disgust over this situation led to countless young people dropping out of society, often banding together on communes or in cooperative housing, and attempting to do their own thing. But one of the difficulties of dropping out is that you've still got to feed yourself, and companies like Kraft and Kellogg's aren't in the business of donating their foods to a bunch of hippies.

And it's not as though the hippies wanted industrially produced food anyway. All big companies, food companies included, were seen as part of the military industrial complex; in other words, the packaged foods sold at supermarkets were the sorts of products that The Man made a profit on. It scarcely mattered whether a company was in the business of manufacturing guns or producing butter: by virtue of it being a large corporation, everything it produced was seen as suspect.

So, in order to feed themselves, America's young dropouts initiated a back-to-the-land movement. Many sought to grow their own food, while others participated in food cooperatives. These co-ops didn't sell products like Pop-Tarts and TV dinners, since that stuff was distrusted. Instead, the foods they offered came in the form of burlap bags filled with rice, grains, and beans.

By purchasing food in this way, the hippies could stick it to the man by bypassing the big food companies. Just as importantly, co-ops enabled people to eat well for a tiny fraction of what it cost to buy processed food at a supermarket. Co-ops offered still another advantage: the foods they sold tended to be far more healthful than the boxed and processed and overly packaged foods created by the big food conglomerates.

Why was this sort of food healthier? Much of the reason was that the food was unadulterated. You were simply buying rice, or potatoes, or soybeans. There weren't 38 ingredients in a given food, nor was there a preservative or artificial coloring anywhere to be found. But probably the most important reason why this food was superior was that it arrived in whole form. The potatoes hadn't been peeled. The rice and wheat didn't have its bran and germ—the healthiest part—milled away. The beans came dry, not in a can with sugar and chunks of factory farmed pig fat.

In other words, the stuff the hippies were buying through their co-ops wasn't *processed food*, it was *whole food*. And the concept of buying—and eating—food in its whole form made too much sense to remain solely in the hands of a bunch of hippies.

Some of the more industrious hippies of that era started food companies geared towards producing this sort of food—packaged, yes, but without the preservatives, without the milling away of vital nutrients, and without the addition of weird colorings and artificial flavorings. By the 1990s, many of these idealistic companies had grown into major food manufacturers, and were bought—you guessed it—by America's top food conglomerates.

Other hippies of that era, most notably Mollie Katzen, wrote cookbooks that sought to offer people methods to prepare these sorts of unprocessed foods in a palatable way.

So within just a couple of decades of the Vietnam war's ending, the key concept that underlay the hippies' style of eating had become thoroughly mainstream. What's more, it had become disproportionately embraced by the most educated and upwardly mobile members of society. Whole Foods Market, for instance, came on the scene and carved out an immensely profitable segment within the grocery industry by specializing in selling the sorts of foods that were based on the hippie philosophy of food production. The genius of Whole Foods Market was in realizing that there were billions of dollars to be made by marketing hippie food to yuppies.

The reason for the spread of counterculture eating is that the underlying philosophy of purchasing whole foods makes too much sense to ignore. You can eat better, cheaper, and more environmentally sustainably by making a point of selecting whole foods, or foods that have been minimally processed.

So, with all of this understood, why should hippies have all the fun? Here's how to incorporate as many whole foods into your diet as possible.

First, buy as much food as you can from your local farmers' markets. Every fruit and vegetable you buy will have been grown locally, and much of it is organic. And, in the spirit of the 1960s counterculture, you've cut out The Man by buying directly from the farmer. By removing the supermarket from the equation, you're buying the freshest possible foods and saving money in the process.

Second, when you do shop at a conventional market, whether it's a natural food store or a regular supermarket, make a habit of looking in your cart as you approach the register. What percentage of your purchases are processed foods in boxes and cans? Hopefully, most of what you're buying are fruits and vegetables, plus bagged grains, rice, nuts, and beans from the bulk department. Make a point of loading up on whole foods like these during your trips to the market. There have been times that I've approached the cash register, looked down into my cart, and noticed that processed foods far outnumbered fresh produce and other whole foods. I've actually turned back from the register in shame and wheeled my cart straight to the produce section to make amends.

One final tip: when you do buy packaged foods, always read the ingredients. Check to see that any grains in the product are in whole form. Avoid colorings, preservatives, artificial flavorings, and anything that just seems like it's not real food.

Eating like a hippie has numerous advantages. It's best for your health, for your wallet, for the planet, and for your transition toward a healthy vegan diet. In fact, once you embrace the counterculture approach to eating, you'll find your resultant food choices will enable you to move more quickly and healthfully to a vegan lifestyle.

I've now finished covering the preliminary information and strategies for transitioning your diet. With this introductory material out of the way, we'll next turn to food shopping and preparation, as well as your various options for dining out. The information I'm about to cover isn't just fun and easy to learn, it will also help you to dramatically accelerate your transition to a vegan diet.

Chapter 11

Supermarket Survival

In Chapter 9, I pointed out that anytime you want, you can pick up the pace in your transition to a vegan diet. With that in mind, by far the best way to speed up your progress is to increase the amount of unfamiliar foods you're sampling each day. Every time you discover a new food you like, it crowds out more of the non-vegan foods you grew up eating.

In this and the next several chapters, I'll be revealing all sorts of strategies for enlarging the variety of vegan foods you enjoy. This chapter is devoted to the very worst place to buy vegan food—your local supermarket. Whenever possible, I recommend buying food at farmers' markets, natural food stores, or online. But there may still be times when it makes sense to visit your local supermarket, and this chapter will help you get the most out of your supermarket visits.

My motto for supermarkets is: so much food, so little to eat. The vast majority of what supermarkets sell is not vegan, and in fact most of the stuff they sell is pure garbage.

The main reason I dislike supermarkets is that they aren't in the business of catering to people like you and me. So, when they do stock healthy vegan foods, they tend to charge outrageous prices. For any given vegan product, supermarkets will often charge nearly double the price that you could find elsewhere.

Really, there are only two good reasons to visit a supermarket: one is if you simply don't have a natural foods store near you, and can't order food online. And the other reason is to take advantage of the produce section—these days, most supermarkets have an excellent produce section and they usually also stock a decent variety of organic produce. And when supermarkets have sales on produce, the prices are often the best you'll find anywhere. I'll sometimes go into a supermarket and buy several pounds of whatever peak-of-season produce item is on sale, and that will be the only purchase I will make.

Let's now check out the remainder of a typical supermarket. I'll guide you through the vegan options that exist in each section.

- **Breads.** This aisle is usually a disappointment. It'll be national brands such as Arnold, Oroweat, and Wonder. The whole wheat bread will usually contain milk products or honey. But better supermarkets will also stock bread from a local bakery. You'll have to check the ingredients, but locally baked bread is frequently vegan. Oddly, these local breads are often kept in a different aisle than the national brands.

  Don't confuse breads baked locally with the supermarket's in-house bakery, where they typically bake some of the nastiest bread ever produced—check the ingredients and you'll see what I'm talking about.

- **Juices.** Some juices are sold on the shelf and others are located in the refrigerated section. Always check the label, since some of these products, particularly smoothies, may contain dairy or honey.

- **Ethnic Foods.** Here, you can find some useful stuff mixed among the menudo and fish flakes. The main vegan foods you can buy here are tamari, noodles, hot sauce, corn and wheat tortillas, and canned chipotles. This section is often adjacent to the rice aisle, which will stock several varieties of brown and white rice in bags. You'll save a lot of money buying your rice in large bags rather than in tiny boxes. You'll also be able to find several kinds of bagged dried beans, from pintos to lentils to split peas.

- **Pasta and Sauces.** Supermarkets carry a wide variety of pasta and noodles. Spaghetti-style pasta is nearly always vegan, and you can also usually find brands made from whole grain. While I love most whole grain breads, some brands of whole grain pasta are terrible—so buy just one package to start to see if you like that particular brand.

  I'll never understand why tomato sauce is so overpriced at supermarkets. You can usually buy organic sauces at your local natural food store for the same price that supermarkets sell their conventional brands. If your supermarket does carry organic sauce, the markup is usually extreme.

- **Condiments.** Nothing too exciting here, but there are plenty of vegan items: ketchup, mustard, olives, pimentos, and tabasco sauce.

- **Flour.** You can of course buy various sorts of flour in the baking aisle, but if you find any baking mixes that are vegan it'll be a minor miracle.

- **Nuts.** Every supermarket sells a good selection of most nuts, as well as sunflower and pumpkin seeds. Watch out for gelatin as an ingredient, which is sometimes added for the sole purpose of annoying vegans. Gelatin is a protein obtained from slaughterhouses.

- **Cereals.** This aisle is surprisingly disappointing. Oddly, most national brands of cereal are scarcely cheaper than organic brands sold at natural food stores. Still, if you read labels, you'll surely find brands of cereal that are free of animal products.

- **Jams, Preserves, and Nut Butters.** You'll find a great selection here, some of which may be organic. Buy jam and preserves instead of jellies, as jellies are mostly sugar.

- **Coffee and Tea.** Better supermarkets will sell fair trade coffee and even have a commercial grade coffee grinder so you can buy whole coffee beans and grind them on the spot.

- **Cookies and Crackers.** The cookie aisle is generally terrible. You're unlikely to find anything that's vegan. You'll do scarcely better in the cracker section. Most items will be non-vegan national brands. But if you look around you can probably find some sort of vegan whole grain cracker. Many varieties of Wasa Crispbread—a European product sold in the cracker aisle, are vegan.

- **Chips and Dips.** Nearly all unflavored potato chips and corn chips are vegan, but check the label to be sure. Stay away from chips made with partially hydrogenated oils, as that stuff is horrible for you. And in the Pennsylvania area, some potato chips are—believe it or not—fried in tallow or lard. Nearly all brands of salsa are vegan. And, increasingly, supermarkets sell refrigerated guacamole in pressure packed boxes. Make sure any guacamole you buy is pressure packed and not just tubbed, as the pressure packed stuff can be excellent, sometimes even better than what you can make at home.

- **Dairy Section.** Most supermarkets carry soymilk packaged in half-gallon milk cartons. Also, calcium-fortified orange juice contains as much calcium as milk, and its calcium is easily absorbed.

- **Frozen Foods.** Amid the salisbury steak TV dinners, there are some surprisingly good vegan options sold in a supermarket's frozen food section. You'll find frozen veggies that are much, much better than canned. You can also buy frozen berries, which are cheap, high quality, and perfect for smoothies (I devote much of chapter 21 to smoothies.) Frozen fruits and veggies are a fantastic option in the dead of winter when good fresh produce isn't widely available. While browsing the frozen foods section, you may also find eggless waffles, veggieburgers, vegan ice creams, and sorbet.

- **Alcohol.** If your state permits supermarkets to sell beer and wine, you can find plenty of vegan brands. Check Appendix C, or the booze list at barnivore.com, to learn which brands of beer and wine are vegan.

As this chapter makes clear, supermarkets offer some good stuff but they scatter it at random throughout the store, leaving it your job to ferret it out. Happily, many supermarkets are setting up aisles and even mini-stores devoted specifically to natural foods. Unfortunately, I've found that there are few bargains to be had in the natural foods sections of supermarkets.

While supermarkets can be a viable source for vegan foods, you'll generally find better prices and a much better selection by taking your business elsewhere. Let's now turn to natural food stores, online shopping options, and farmers' markets.

Chapter 12

Natural Food Stores

Now that we've considered your vegan options in supermarkets, it's time to give the same treatment to natural food stores.

When you're checking out a natural food store, the first thing you need to do is to determine if it's any good. That's because there are really two kinds of natural food stores: bad ones and good ones. The bad natural food stores aren't really natural food stores at all—they're just glorified vitamin shops that carry a paltry selection of overpriced food. These places aren't worth your time and money.

Fortunately, there's an easy way to distinguish a good natural food store from a bad one: just check the produce section. Some of these stores don't even carry produce, while others make a pathetic and half-hearted attempt to stock some bananas and apples. If the place isn't willing to sell fruits and vegetables, you can bet they are making nearly all their money on selling vitamins. What you have is not a food store, it's a pill store! You'll do ten times better shopping for food anyplace else, including a regular supermarket.

But a *good* natural food store, one that's actually in the business of selling food, offers an entirely different experience. There, you'll find great produce, with many more organic items than a regular supermarket would sell. And you'll find tons of vegan products that aren't available elsewhere.

You may already know where the natural food stores are in your town. If not, they are easy to find. Just check the yellow pages under groceries and there ought to be a natural foods or health foods subheading. Also, visit WholeFoodsMarket.com and TraderJoes.com. These websites will enable you to find out if these vegan-friendly chains have stores in your area.

Where natural food markets are concerned, bigger is often better. The more floor space they have, the more different sorts of vegan goodies you can buy. Since the selection of vegan foods is so much better than what a typical supermarket will stock, I can't take you through the store section-by-section like I did in the preceding chapter on supermarkets—there's just too much to cover.

Instead, let me tell you about a few key areas to focus on. The better stores feature delis offering freshly-made food. Usually this stuff is quite expensive, but if you're new to veganism I recommend you buy four or five of the most appealing items anyway. Why? Because if there's a single piece of advice I keep coming back to, it's that the speed at which you can comfortably transition to a vegan diet depends on the rate at which you try new foods. A natural foods deli is a great way to get several new foods under your belt without investing any real time or effort. What's more, most of the foods sold in a deli turn out to be fairly easy to prepare. So if you fall in love with the tabouli, or the peanut lime Asian noodles, it's a simple matter to track down a recipe, or just wing it based on the ingredients the dish contains.

Next up, let's look at the refrigerated section. There, you'll find all sorts of things you can't find at your supermarket or online. If you live in a progressive, veggie friendly city, you'll find a number of terrific pre-made items produced by local companies. The only things I'd advise against buying are the sandwiches, as they tend to be inexplicably expensive, and it's never good to let bread sit for hours or days after a sandwich is made.

The refrigerated section will also feature several kinds of fake meat, as well as vegan cheeses, yogurts, and mayonnaise. This section should also carry tofu, tempeh, and seitan—these foods are featured in a number of recipes, and stick to your ribs the way meat does. Finally, look for fresh eggless pasta, which, although expensive, tastes infinitely better than dried pasta.

Now let's leave the refrigerated section and visit the area where a good natural food store really shines: the bulk foods department. Here we'll find pasta, dried beans, rice, grains, numerous varieties of flour, and a wide assortment of nuts and dried fruit. If that's not enough, you can even find some fantastic vegan candy: many places will carry chocolate coconut haystacks that are vegan and ridiculously good. Some bulk departments will also sell various nut butters, which you'll scoop straight from the bucket into your own container. And don't forget that bulk departments usually offer spices and coffee in bulk as well. The spices in particular are generally sold at a huge discount over pre-packaged brands.

I always hit the frozen foods section last since I don't want these foods to melt during the trip home. But if you're on a budget, I recommend avoiding all frozen foods except berries and veggies. Whereas non-vegan frozen foods can be extremely cheap, vegan frozen foods are often a budget buster. Whether we're talking pizza or pot pies or frozen entrees, the cost of these items frequently borders on exorbitant, and the serving sizes tend to be tiny.

Still, you can find some interesting foods in the frozen section, and just looking at the packaging may give you an idea of things you want to cook from scratch. Plus, there are several excellent brands of vegan ice cream. These ice creams vary considerably from one brand to the next, so try them all in order to decide which ones you like best.

The cereal, crackers, chips, and cookies aisles will look a lot like that of a typical supermarket. But the products will tend to be made from better ingredients, more expensive, and much more likely to be vegan.

Before you leave the store, remember that it's all about the produce. So, unless you are a regular at your local farmers' market, be sure to load up your cart with fruits and veggies.

Chapter 13

Farmers' Markets

Farmers' markets have it all. They are outdoors in the fresh air. They offer tons of sustainably grown, organic, local produce. And nearly everything they sell has been picked that same morning. So if there's a farmers' market near you, and you're not regularly shopping there, you are missing out on all sorts of great foods.

It's easy to find farmers' markets in your area: Localharvest.org lists most of the farmers' markets in the United States. In California and in southern states, many farmers' markets operate year-round. In colder regions, these markets may only be open three to six months per year. Most farmers' markets are open for just a few hours one or two days a week.

To get the most out of farmers' markets, you need to adjust your style of shopping. In a regular grocery store, you walk in and see some beautiful ripe peaches at a decent price, so you load up your basket and everything is right in the world. But do the same thing at a farmers' market and the situation will play out differently. Suppose you see some gorgeous peaches for a reasonable price, so you go ahead and make your purchase. What will happen next is you'll get halfway through the market and see another farmer selling even more beautiful peaches, plus they're organic, and for fifty cents a pound less. Well, you've already bought peaches from the first vendor, so you're all peached out.

The lesson here is that you should never, ever, make a single purchase at a farmers' market before completing a quick walk-through to see what each vendor carries. The heartbreak of buying something and then encountering the very same item nicer and cheaper just a few stalls down will haunt you until your dying day.

One of my favorite things about farmers' markets is that each table is typically staffed by somebody from the farm, who works at the crops nearly every day. They'll be able to tell you exactly how the mustard greens crop is shaping up, or whether they think the raspberry harvest will last into next week's market. Over time you get to know them and they get to know you—and suddenly you've got a genuine connection to your food supply. These people also tend to be some of the nicest folks you'll ever meet. When I lived in Berkeley I used to love hitting the farmers' market there; I'd always have a little chat with this older grape farmer who showed up in a beat-up red 1950s Ford pickup truck. The guy looked a bit like Santa but he'd have these stories of how he used to race motorcycles. He'd always come with at least five different varieties of grapes, all hand-picked by him that morning; how could buying grapes at a supermarket compare?

And let's not forget the prepared vegan food that is often available at these markets. Some of the best food I've ever eaten has come from farmers' markets stalls: a fantastic macrobiotic platter in central New York, incredible Middle Eastern food at the Hollywood farmers' market, and tandoori-baked flatbread in Santa Cruz. Not every farmers' market offers food like this, but it's surprising how many vegan-friendly food businesses manage to get stalls at their local markets. I often convince myself that I'm going to the farmers' market to buy my kale and potatoes for the week, but I suspect the real reason I'm going is because I'm Jonesing for some of those fresh-from-the-deep-fryer corn fritters I can't get anyplace else.

I hope this brief chapter conveys the mellow vibe that descends on every farmers' market. Yeah, you're typically in a bit of a crowd, but it's a relaxed and happy crowd, buying fantastic stuff that's overwhelmingly vegan. How could you not be happy too?

There is also a close cousin of a farmers' market known as a CSA, which stands for Community Supported Agriculture. Here, you buy a share of a given farm's output for a season, and once a week you go to a drop-off point to pick up your box of goodies. Alternately, some CSAs deliver right to your doorstep.

CSAs are wonderful because they guarantee your farmer a steady income for the season, and these arrangements can go a long way toward making a farm that's local to you economically viable. The same website I mentioned at the start of this chapter, localharvest.org, also maintains a listing of CSAs.

It's a lot easier to eat plenty of fruits and veggies when you're buying the freshest, cheapest, and most local stuff available. And if you're ever strolling through your local farmers' market and have a UVO sighting—an Unidentified Vegetable Object—I urge you to find out what it's called, buy it, and check your cookbooks or the Internet for a way to prepare it.

So take your time while visiting your farmers' market. Stroll around. Enjoy the fresh air. Linger a little longer than necessary at each table, and make a point of buying those cute little peppers or those thick fragrant leeks. Life is more than taking time to smell the roses, it's also about knocking on the watermelon to test its ripeness, and sniffing the cilantro. Short of doing your own gardening, nothing gets you closer to the moment of harvest than a visit to your local farmers' market.

Chapter **14**

Online Groceries

Not so long ago, shopping for vegan food online was prohibitively expensive. When the Web got popular in the late 1990s, a number of vegan specialty merchants quickly set up shop. Many of these businesses still exist today. Some of these companies are essentially one-stop online department stores featuring items like vegan shoes, candles, marshmallows, and so forth. Other websites are run by vegan bakeries, and sell cookies and other treats by mail.

These sorts of websites are useful for specialty items, but none of these companies seem to be in the business of selling everyday vegan grocery items at a reasonable price. In most cases, shipping costs alone make these independent sites too expensive to compete with your local food retailers.

Happily, this situation changed when Amazon.com decided to get into the grocery business. True, most of Amazon's grocery selection isn't vegan. But they do carry hundreds of great vegan products, often at highly competitive prices. In fact, for some categories such as energy bars, you'd be hard-pressed to find an equivalent selection in your community. Add to this the fact that Amazon offers free shipping on the grocery products it directly fulfills, and their offerings become hard to beat.

For several items including energy bars, cookies, salad dressing, and vitamins, I personally wouldn't shop anywhere but Amazon. But again, there's the problem that all this great vegan stuff is buried under a mountain of non-vegan items. And, as of this writing, Amazon really doesn't offer a convenient way for customers to filter out its non-vegan offerings.[1]

Amazon of course doesn't offer any fresh veggies, nor does it sell items that require refrigeration. But for a number of shelf-stable vegan food products, the company offers unbeatable prices and selection.

---

[1] At Vegan.com, I've set up an online store devoted to Amazon's vegan offerings. You can visit this store at:

http://grocery.vegan.com/

Disclosure: purchases made through Vegan.com generate commissions that I use to keep the site running. If you already know exactly what you want to purchase, it's just as easy to go directly through Amazon's main page, since there is no difference in price or selection.

Chapter 15

Non-Vegetarian Restaurants

We just spent the past several chapters exploring supermarkets, natural food stores, farmers' markets, and online retailers. After all that exhausting shopping, it's time to sit down, relax, and let somebody else do the cooking. So in this chapter and the one that follows, we're going to check out the vegan options that exist in restaurants.

This chapter is devoted to non-vegetarian restaurants, and how to know in advance which of these places are reasonably vegan-friendly. I will also cover which common restaurant foods are least likely to contain animal products.

Non-vegetarian restaurants can be quite accommodating to vegans. So let's begin by looking at the least appealing options of all, just so we can get them out of the way.

Subway offers salads and the erroneously named Veggie Delight sandwich. If you do decide to purchase the Veggie Delight, be sure to have them hold the cheese and the mayo. Plus, you've got to order it on white bread if you want to avoid the honey. This is one of the most boring sandwiches ever made; iceberg lettuce anyone? And the fact that it's almost as expensive as their meat-based sandwiches is totally unfair. But with nearly 30,000 locations worldwide, it's never hard to find a Subway, and so a Veggie Delight can be an OK option if nothing else is available. When driving long distances, it's good to know that there's a Subway on the Interstate every twenty miles or so, and that you can therefore reliably get vegan food without any advance planning. One final point about Subway, though: the knife they use to cut the sandwich in half is an entity of supreme nastiness, since it cuts hundreds of meat sandwiches a day and they never seem to clean it. So on the rare occasions that I eat at Subway, I always ask them not to cut my sandwich in two.

Taco Bell is another option, I guess. There, you can get a bean tostada, or a bean burrito hold the cheese. Unlike Subway, where you can see your sandwich being made and let out a scream if they're about to squirt on mayonnaise, the Taco Bell stuff is made back in the kitchen. The incompetence of Taco Bell's food preparers is the stuff of legends. Let's just say that if Taco Bell ever decides to do drug testing, they'll have to fire half their workforce.

So never bite into a Taco Bell burrito without first opening it up to see if there is some evil animal product lurking within. I really can't recommend Taco Bell under any circumstances. It's one of those places where you arrive hungry and leave feeling bloated and drugged. What a brothel is to love, Taco Bell is to food—although I must admit that in the 1970s, I used to love the fake bell that adorned each restaurant's roof. Those were cool.

Now that we've gotten Subway and Taco Bell out of the way, the chain options improve enormously. P.F. Chang's Bistro is a terrific Chinese-style restaurant with lots of vegan stuff on the menu. In fact, every option in the "Vegetarian Plates and Sides" section of their menu is vegan. Note that most of this stuff contains cane sugar, which may be filtered through bone char. But I don't consider this an issue worth paying attention to—Chapter 24 explains my take on animal ingredients.

The amazing thing about P.F. Chang's is that the décor is surprisingly swanky, yet it's impossible for any one person to eat more than about $15 worth of food. Nearly all of P.F. Chang's offerings are veggie-based stir-fry dishes, and they do an amazing job with eggplant as well. They've got more than 130 restaurants in the United States, and as full-service chains go, they really can't be beaten.

My two other favorite chain options are Chipotle Mexican Grill and Qdoba. Of the two, I favor Chipotle since they make a real effort to source organic ingredients for their food, plus their chips are sensational. Also, Chipotle consistently serves huge burritos, whereas I've found Qdoba's offerings are sometimes way too small. There's really only one item I recommend at either of these chains, and that's a bean burrito with rice, salsa, and guacamole. If you're at a Chipotle, have them add the grilled peppers, and if you're at a Qdoba, ask for the grilled veggies. Chipotle's corn salsa is also fantastic, and you can ask them to add some hot sauce as well. But make sure you only order black beans at Chipotle restaurants since their pinto beans annoyingly contain pork.

For vegans, both of these chains impose what I call the burrito tax. That is, they charge you the same price as everyone else for a vegetarian burrito, even though you've asked to leave off the cheese and sour cream. It's totally unfair, since you pay what everyone else pays but you get substantially less food, despite the fact that cheese and sour cream are two of a burrito's costliest ingredients.

Now that we've considered chain restaurants, let's take a look at non-vegetarian independent restaurants.

When deciding what sort of independent non-veggie restaurant to patronize, it makes sense to choose by cuisine. Some cuisines are perfect for vegans, while others you should avoid at all costs.

By far the most vegan-friendly cuisine is Middle Eastern,

which sounds like a bizarre thing to say since the the kitchens of these restaurants invariably showcase a revolving hunk of lamb on a spit. The thing is, so long as you're not eating meat, virtually everything else in the restaurant will be vegan. Eggs simply don't show up in Middle Eastern cooking, and dairy products are a rarity. The breads and rices and main entrees, so long as they don't contain meat, are pretty much guaranteed to be vegan. Many Middle Eastern places serve pita bread stuffed with falafel, hummus, or baba ghanouj. You can't go wrong with any of these choices. Alternately, you may be able to order a wrap-style sandwich served in a flatbread called lavash—which I consider a far tastier option than pita bread. And just about every Middle Eastern place will offer a vegetarian plate containing falafel, hummus, baba ghanouj, tabouli, pita, and tahini dressing. In a few falafel joints, most of these actually Greek rather than Middle Eastern, the hummus or the tahini dressing may be adulterated with yogurt, so be sure to ask. Everything else I've just mentioned should always be vegan.

If I can't get Middle Eastern food, my second choice would be Ethiopian. Every Ethiopian restaurant will offer a half-dozen different vegan stews. They'll serve a large dollop of each variety of stew on a giant sour fermented vegan pancake called injera bread. Typically, this will be served family style, with your dinner companions gathered around, tearing off pieces of injera, and dipping it into the various stews. A small percentage of Ethiopian restaurants cook using clarified butter, or kibur, so call ahead to ask. But since vegetable oil is so inexpensive, nearly all Ethiopian restaurants cook without butter. Ethiopian restaurants may occasionally plop a dollop of sour cream at the center of the meal as a garnish, so be sure to specify that you don't eat dairy products.

If you can't get Middle Eastern or Ethiopian food, after that the drop-off gets pretty severe. You can go to a sushi place and order pretty much anything featuring seaweed, rice, and veggies. Just be sure to say you don't eat eggs, and, of course, fish. Vegan sushi is fantastic, one of my favorite things to eat in fact. But you're always better off making it yourself, since sushi restaurants usually charge vegans fish prices to eat a bunch of rice and veggies. And besides, making sushi at home is fun and easy, and you can use a better and fresher selection of veggies than any sushi restaurant will offer.

Mexican food can be workable, but it's a minefield. You have to watch out for chicken stock in the rice, and occasionally lard in the tortillas. The guacamole may be vegan, or it may contain sour cream. Order your beans whole instead of refried, unless you're sure that the refried beans are made without lard. Many Mexican restaurants warm their tortillas on the same grill on which they cook their meats.

If you're in the mood for a light meal, a freshly-baked bagel can be a nice choice. Unfortunately, while bagels made from white flour will nearly always be vegan, whole wheat bagels often contain honey. If you're lucky, your bagel place can add some hummus, sprouts, and tomatoes and suddenly you've got a legitimate vegan meal.

I suppose you could always hit a salad bar, but those places consistently disappoint and annoy me. I mean, you would think a salad bar would be a vegan paradise. But the soups won't be vegan, the muffins and breads won't be vegan, and the dessert options won't be vegan either. On top of all that, you're even shafted with your choice of dressings—pretty much your only vegan options for dressing will be oil and vinegar or Italian. I get angry just thinking about it. Let's move on.

Scraping the bottom of the barrel, you could always get a cheeseless pizza. Unfortunately, many of the big chains put dairy products in their dough. Luckily, an authentic neighborhood-style pizzeria will make their dough from scratch, with just flour, yeast, water, sugar, and salt. And the sauce will be vegan too. Just keep in mind that many pizzerias dust their pies with parmesan, so be sure to ask for no cheese at all, including no parmesan—claim a dairy allergy if you must. As with the burrito tax I mentioned earlier, you're generally stuck paying for a cheese-bearing pie even though the most expensive ingredient is being left off.

Since we are now nearly out of options, I'll finish by telling you the restaurants I avoid at all costs. I generally don't do Indian at all, unless I know for sure that the place goes out of its way to cater to vegans. Dairy shows up in way too much Indian food and is often undetectable what with all the spices.

And you can forget about Chinese food, with the exception of P.F. Chang's. At most non-vegetarian Chinese restaurants, chicken stock can be in practically anything, and you'll never know.

There are of course dozens of other restaurant chains that I don't have room to cover in this chapter. Fortunately, there's a website, VeganEatingOut.com, that brings together current vegan-oriented information for every major restaurant chain in America. So if you're ever stuck attending a gathering at Applebee's or T.G.I. Friday's, you can check VeganEatingOut.com beforehand to find out just how shafted you really are.

Your best bet, of course, is not to go to a single restaurant I've mentioned in this chapter. If at all possible, I patronize vegan places. I favor vegan restaurants because I like to be certain that my food is vegan, and also because it's important to keep money within the veggie community. As we're about to see, there are some truly amazing all-veggie restaurants out there for you to enjoy, with more of these restaurants opening every year.

Chapter **16**

Veggie Restaurants

Now that we've looked at non-vegetarian restaurants, it's time
to consider veggie restaurants. While I don't have much to say
in this chapter, I think that what little advice I can provide here
will be extremely useful.

Thanks to the Internet, it's easy to find veggie restaurants
in your vicinity. There are three different websites dedicated to
providing listings and reviews for vegetarian restaurants: Happy-
Cow.net, VegGuide.org, and VegDining.com. All three of these
sites are worth checking out, since you'll find restaurants and
reviews on one that you won't find on the others.

Also, be sure to check out Yelp.com, which is an unbeatable
resource for vegetarians and vegans. Yelp is an incredibly popular
site where people post reviews for every restaurant, business, and
organization in their community. It's astonishing the number of
reviews that you can find through Yelp. Just do a search for
vegan in your zip code, and every restaurant that somebody has
tagged as offering vegan options will come up.

Yelp is one of the handful of gigantic websites that, like Ama-
zon.com or eBay, has reached critical mass. Let me give you an
idea of Yelp's comprehensiveness. There's a veggie restaurant
called Fragrance Land near my parents' house that I always eat

at whenever I'm in town. It's not a well-known restaurant, and had only been around for eighteen months when I looked for it on Yelp. At the time, I doubted whether anyone had yet added it to Yelp's directory. But when I typed *vegan* into Yelp's search box, along with my parents' zip code, Fragrance Land came up as number two on a lengthy list of nearby vegan-friendly restaurants. Here I was wondering if even one person had reviewed the restaurant, and I found 42 different reviews.

So just for the fun of it, I looked up how many Yelp members had posted reviews for San Francisco's Millennium restaurant, which may be the most famous vegan gourmet restaurant in the United States. There were 444 reviews!

No matter what the restaurant, the members of Yelp will give you the inside scoop on the place. After reading the reviews, you'll not only know if a restaurant is worth visiting, you'll also find out what items are not-to-be-missed, and which offerings consistently disappoint. So, just by spending some time on Yelp, you'll find out about all the veggie and veggie-friendly places in your town, and you'll probably know exactly what you want to order before you even look at the menu.

As I said at the start of this chapter, there's not much information I need to provide about veggie restaurants. But I still have a couple more tips to offer. The first is that it's important to distinguish between vegetarian and vegan restaurants. It is incredibly easy to let your guard down regarding dairy and eggs when you're eating at a vegetarian restaurant. You feel like, for once in your life, you're on your home turf, and don't need to be vigilant about asking about the vegan status of your food. Next thing you know, there's cheese garnishing your vegetarian chili, or you've been served a piece of pie that has butter in the crust. Sadly, some veggie restaurants are surprisingly indifferent to adequately taking care of their vegan clientele.

So unless you're eating in a specifically vegan restaurant, it's important not to make any assumptions about the vegan status of your food. It's strange and sad that it takes less effort to be vegan in a traditional Middle Eastern restaurant than it does in a typical ovo-lacto vegetarian restaurant, but that's how it is.

I've got one final piece of advice, and this one's a biggie. It's common for veggie restaurants to offer a hodgepodge of ethnic dishes. Some typical offerings are falafel and hummus, Indian curries, and burritos.

I try to avoid anything from distant cultures when eating at veggie restaurants, unless that restaurant specializes exclusively in that cuisine. That's because the ethnic dishes almost always disappoint. The falafel and hummus will generally be terrible compared to what you can get in an authentic Middle Eastern restaurant. The curry will typically be incompetently spiced and badly prepared. And I'm quite confident that the worst burrito ever made came from a veggie restaurant that also serves entrees adapted from six other cultures. I'm not claiming that my rule applies in every case, but generally the foods from cultures outside your country will be the worst items on the menu. So make your selection with that tendency in mind.

I think this short chapter provided pretty much everything you need to know about eating at veggie restaurants. And since it's always more fun to eat with a group, I highly recommend hitting Meetup.com to see if there are veggie dineouts happening in your area.

Chapter **17**

International Travel

People tend to freak out when confronted with the idea of traveling as a vegan. Happily, with sufficient preparation, it's generally fairly easy to stay vegan while traveling. Few countries are as veggie-friendly as the United States, but with a little planning you can eat well almost anywhere.

If you're considering a trip abroad, the most helpful action I can recommend is to go online and research the vegan possibilities that exist for the country you intend to visit. You'll learn a great deal of helpful information by doing internet searches using the words "vegan," and "vegetarian," plus the city and country you'll be visiting. This sort of simple research can help you discover veggie-friendly restaurants at your destination.

It also makes sense to learn something about the staple foods of whichever country you're visiting. By doing so, you'll learn which foods are dependably vegan, and which dishes to avoid. For instance, no matter where you travel in Mexico or South America, you can be confident that the freshly-made corn tortillas sold by street vendors are always vegan. The more you learn about your destination's cuisine, the easier and more gastronomically fulfilling your visit will be.

Yet all the research in the world won't erase the challenges that accompany visiting a country with limited vegetarian options. One unpleasant travel surprise is that many destinations are still in the dark ages when it comes to vegetarianism. Take Barcelona, Spain, as one example: a beautiful, modern, and comparatively wealthy city that one vegan friend of mine, who has lived there for years, decries as having practically no veggie-friendly restaurants.

Happily, even if your restaurant options are limited, you'll almost certainly have access to markets featuring a wide variety of rices, beans, fruits, nuts, and vegetables. You're also likely to encounter varieties of locally-grown fruits that you can't get at home. For instance, markets in both Hawaii and Central America feature "apple bananas"—bananas about half as long and slightly stouter than the variety typically exported to Western countries. These bananas have a texture, flavor, and tanginess that are vastly superior to the bananas sold in Western supermarkets.

As with any other effort you make in life, it makes sense to focus on the positive. That is, rather than lamenting over the culinary limitations of your destination, you're better off trying to identify the strengths of the local cuisine. In most exotic locales, you'll be able to identify at least a handful of regional specialties that just happen to be vegan—foods you either can't get at home or that, by virtue of their authenticity, blow away the versions you can buy in your own country.

So, under no circumstances should you travel abroad without first exploring online the dining options you'll have available. It's not always easy to be vegan when traveling internationally, but by doing some basic research in advance, you're likely to turn your dining options into a highlight of your trip.

Chapter 18

Convenience Foods

Of all the chapters in this book, this is the one that can push you most rapidly towards becoming vegan. Here, I run through the finest convenience foods I know. If you make a point of trying everything mentioned here, you'll no doubt find several items you'll want to always have on hand.

Stocking your pantry with these convenience foods can make a huge difference in your quality of life. Sometimes you'll suddenly find yourself hungry and want something to eat *right now*, not thirty minutes from now. Luckily, as we're about to see, you've got plenty of vegan options. It's hard to overstate the importance of keeping delicious vegan convenience foods in your pantry at all times. I hope you'll make life easy on yourself and stock up on as many of these foods as possible.

- **Energy Bars.** There are about a dozen different brands of vegan energy bars on the market. Clif Bars are the most popular. They're cheap, made largely from organic ingredients, and are bulky enough to be a substantial snack. My two favorite flavors are Chocolate Chip and Cool Mint Chocolate. I love to smear some organic nut butter on a Chocolate Chip Clif Bar and serve it with a glass of soymilk or almond milk.

Luna Bars are made by the Clif Bar people and are marketed to women. Although it's emasculating to purchase Luna Bars if you're a guy, it's worth the embarrassment because they're really good. They're smaller than Clif Bars, much sweeter, and are coated with chocolate. In contrast to Clif Bars, most flavors of Luna Bars taste pretty similar. There's not a flavor I dislike.

Larabars are another popular energy bar, and they are nothing like Clif or Luna Bars because they are made almost entirely of fruit and nuts. Their Cherry Pie bar is one of my all-time favorite food products. What's astonishing about this offering is how it exactly captures several of the best flavor notes from a cherry pie, despite being a vegan product consisting entirely of dates, almonds, and cherries. I don't know how they managed this: it's like eating a real cherry pie that is somehow good for you.

Finally, you might want to try the energy bars made by ProBar. While they cost more than Clif Bars, ProBars are larger and made from more expensive ingredients. Their flavors and textures are outstanding, perhaps the best of any energy bar.

- **Entrees.** There are numerous brands of boxed Indian-style entrees, made in India and packaged in shelf-stable foil envelopes. This is about as authentically fancy as cheap convenience food can get, and many of these products are vegan. Most natural food stores carry this sort of product under the Tasty Bite label. At Indian groceries, you'll find a half-dozen other brands. Depending on the brand and the variety, these products range from scarcely edible to sublime—the best brand I've tried is Kitchens of India. Always check the ingredients before making a purchase as only about 30 percent of the products in this category are vegan.

These Indian entrees are best served over rice—but what's the point of having an instant entree like this if your rice needs thirty minutes to cook? Here, Trader Joe's comes to the rescue by selling pre-cooked brown rice that requires only a minute in the microwave.

Another great entree to serve over pre-cooked brown rice is canned vegan chili. There are several brands available: Amy's is especially good.

- **Chips.** Kettle Chips is probably the best-known producer of premium potato chips, and many of their potato chip flavors are vegan.

I think potato chips are overrated. What I really miss from my pre-vegan days were those poofy cheese puffs with the bright orange "cheeze" powder that would get all over your hands. Happily, the vegan world has a delicious counterpart to that nutritional travesty: Tings. They're crisp, light, and have that same salty crunch. Marvelous.

Tortilla chips are another fine junk food. Plus you can dip them into salsa, so even if the chips themselves are oily and salty, at least they're carrying along some great nutrition. On the rare occasions when I eat corn chips, I prefer the ones made from blue corn.

- **Crackers.** In Chapter 11, I was pessimistic about your prospects for finding decent crackers in the supermarket. Fortunately, there are sensational vegan crackers available elsewhere. One product I often eat is Late July peanut butter sandwich crackers. These crackers evoke all sorts of nostalgic childhood feelings for me of those peanut butter sandwich crackers I ate as a kid. Yet they're vegan and far healthier, since they're made with all-organic ingredients.

Best of all, they're about the same price as the cruddy nonvegan crackers that supermarkets sell. You can find these crackers at natural food stores and online.

- **Cookies.** Nana's makes oversized inexpensive vegan cookies. It's incredibly difficult to make a tasty mass-produced cookie without resorting to white flour, yet Nana's has managed to do it. And their flour isn't just whole-grain, it's organic too. They've also got several varieties that are either wheat or gluten free. By weight, they're cheaper than most energy bars, and they don't have any refined sugar either. Nana's aren't the best vegan cookies I've ever had, but they're pretty darn good, and I always keep some in my kitchen cupboard. All the flavors are tasty, and my favorite is coconut chip. Amazon.com carries these at a great price, and many natural food stores stock them as well.

  Much less healthy are the bagged vegan cookies sold by Trader Joe's. The chocolate chip flavor is remarkable, and your friends won't believe they're vegan.

  The best commercially made vegan cookies I've ever had are from Allison's Gourmet and Liz Lovely. Allison's is available from the company website (allisonsgourmet.com), while Liz Lovely is available online (lizlovely.com), and at natural food stores on the East Coast and Central United States.

There are probably a hundred other great vegan convenience foods in addition to those I've covered in this brief chapter, and new products are being dreamed up all the time. So, no doubt, you'll end up with some favorites not mentioned here. But the items presented in this chapter are widely loved by the vegan community, and should be more than sufficient to get you started.

Chapter **19**

Meat, Dairy, & Egg Replacements

When the subject of veganism comes up, omnivores often say, "I could never give up cheese," or, "I like a good steak now and then."

So in this chapter, we will go through the main sorts of animal products that people eat, and we will consider the vegan replacements that exist. Some of the vegan foods we'll look at are either indistinguishable from the non-vegan foods they replace, or are close enough that it hardly matters. The best brands of vegan mayonnaise, ice cream sandwiches, soy yogurt, and ground meat substitutes fall into this category.

We'll also look at some vegan foods that bear only the slightest resemblance to the non-vegan foods they replace, but are still wonderfully tasty items in their own right. In fact, you might end up liking some of these foods much more than the animal products you formerly ate. Two of these not-even-close yet delicious replacements are sautéed portobello mushrooms instead of hamburgers and scrambled tofu instead of scrambled eggs.

While I think there are tons of fantastic items that can satisfy your cravings for meat, milk, and eggs, I'm not going to suggest that every such substitute is wonderful. In fact, some meat and cheese replacements are simply disgusting. Back in the 1980s, many of the meat and cheese substitutes on the market were simply terrible; a culinary assault on the tastebuds. Happily, today there is too much competition in the vegan marketplace for inferior foods to survive.

So now let's consider some great replacements for meat, dairy, and egg-based foods.

Meat

I once had a conversation about meat substitutes with Jennifer Raymond, one of the most successful vegan cookbook authors of the 1990s. She told me:

> If somebody likes the textures, flavors, and the spices that are commonly associated with meat, I can give them vegan foods that have all these things. But if that person insists on the experience of eating a T-bone steak, well then they're out of luck. There's nothing in the vegan world that will replicate an intact piece of cow muscle.

It's been nearly a decade since I had that conversation with Jennifer, and in that time the fake meat options have only gotten better. While there's still nothing at all like a T-bone steak, there are now some exceptional vegan meat replacements. My favorite brand is the ground meat and seafood products made by Match Premium Vegan Meats. These are not yet distributed nationally, but you can order them directly through MatchMeats.com. The ground beef, pork, and chicken versions of their products are note-perfect replacements for meat—they could absolutely fool a meat eater.

Comparably great are the sausages and related products created by the Field Roast Grain Meat Company. These are distributed to natural food stores throughout the United States. I consider their Celebration Loaf to be the centerpiece for the best Thanksgiving-style vegan dinner you could possibly serve.

Tofurky brand sausages are also good, with the Italian style being their best offering. Every once in a while, I like to go all-out cooking on a weekend morning: fried potatoes, sautéed kale, pancakes, and sliced and pan-fried sausages from either Field Roast or Tofurky make for the ultimate vegan brunch.

Let's now turn to meat substitutes that won't fool anyone, but can be delicious in their own way. My favorite of these is falafel, which I've talked about earlier in this book. Falafel is a Middle Eastern deep-fried meatball made from chick peas, garlic, and parsley. Served in pita bread with some veggies and tahini sauce, you've got something way tastier than any burger.

Another delicious meaty sandwich is made from pan-fried portobello mushrooms. Just remove the woody, inedible stem and fry each side of the cap in a bit of oil over medium heat for a minute or two, then serve it on a hamburger bun with all the fixings. These mushrooms happen to be exactly the size of a large hamburger patty.

There are a number of dishes where you'll want the chewy texture of meat, but don't really need meat's flavor. For this sort of thing, frozen tofu is hard to beat. Just buy a package of tofu, cut it into slices, then freeze the slices overnight. The freezing will dramatically change the tofu's texture, giving it a meaty chewiness. And since nothing compares to tofu in terms of soaking up surrounding flavors, this is a terrific choice for use in dishes that have spicy, rich, or flavorful sauces. Slices of frozen tofu, cut into small pieces, are outstanding when added to vegan chili.

As with frozen tofu, tempeh is another great choice to lend a meaty texture to a vegan dish. Nearly all vegan cookbooks feature a few tempeh recipes, so give one of these recipes a try.

Dairy Products

Let's cover the best dairy alternatives first: there are vegan brands of ice cream and yogurt that are incredible. Specifically, the vegan ice creams made by So Delicious and Double Rainbow are to-die-for. The best thing So Delicious makes is their coconut-based ice-cream. Double Rainbow makes both dairy and vegan ice creams—their Very Cherry Chocolate Chip flavor is magnificent. Trader Joe's sells this product at a fantastic price under their own private label brand. Finally, WholeSoy makes a frozen soy yogurt that contains about half the calories of vegan ice cream, yet offers exceptional flavor.

When it comes to soy yogurt, I don't know of a bad brand. I think that when yogurt bacteria go to work, the sour flavors produced become dominant and so the yogurt's flavor doesn't differ by much whether the base ingredient is cow's milk or soymilk. I can strongly recommend any of these brands: White Wave, So Delicious, Silk, and Wildwood. Nancy's, a company known mainly for dairy-based yogurts, also makes a line of excellent soy yogurts—and after years of complaints from vegans they finally responded and got rid of the honey.

Ten or twenty years ago, just about every brand of vegan cheese was a grotesque abomination. You'd heat it in the oven and it wouldn't actually melt. If you were lucky, it would start perspiring and soften to a plasticky texture. The stuff tasted horrible and would seemingly sit in your stomach for days without digesting.

Today, most brands of vegan cheeses are at least tolerable, but you've still got to be careful when purchasing the stuff. Always check the label for casein, or some chemical with casein as part of its name. Casein is a milk protein, and unfortunately several companies manufacture casein-based soy cheeses without disclosing on the label that this ingredient comes from milk.

I rarely eat commercially-produced vegan cheese, but I do like to use it for the occasional grilled cheese sandwich. My favorite type of vegan cheese is the one I make myself. Appendix D contains my recipe for cashew cheese, which I think makes a delicious pizza topping. I've been getting requests for this recipe ever since I mentioned it in my first book.

One final recommendation where cheese is concerned: there are vegan brands of cream cheese that are surprisingly good. Lightly toasted raisin bread with vegan cream cheese, sprouts, and chopped walnuts is one of my favorite treats.

It's funny that so many potential vegans fret about giving up cheese, yet I don't think I've ever heard a single person voice misgivings about giving up milk. The reason, I think, is that most people don't terribly enjoy the flavor of milk. In fact, most vegans end up saying they strongly prefer the flavor of soy, rice, or almond milk to anything that comes out of Bessie's mammary glands.

Admittedly, milk does excel in coffee. Regular soymilk does not blend into coffee the way milk does. And, of course, many coffee drinkers really want cream or at least half-and-half in their coffee. Some coffee drinkers will view a switch to soymilk as perfectly fine, while others will count it as a heavy blow. Fortunately, Silk makes a product especially for coffee that blends like cream and carries a rich and pleasant taste—this "Silk Creamer" product comes in three flavors.

Let's end this section on dairy products with a mention of butter. Earth Balance has a stranglehold on the vegan butter market, and for good reason. The stuff is cheap and delicious, and there's even an organic whipped version. But I'd lose all credibility if I tried to claim that Earth Balance is the flavor equal of real butter. Butter simply has some delicate flavor notes that may never be perfectly captured in a soy-based product. That said, in many recipes, you won't taste the difference by using Earth Balance.

Eggs

For their binding and moistening properties, many people consider eggs to be an essential ingredient for baked desserts. Fortunately, nothing could be further from the truth. Anyone suffi-
ciently knowledgeable about how to use ingredients like ground
flax, apple sauce, and tapioca will lose no kitchen powers by
swearing off eggs. And for general baking use, a widely-available
product called, sensibly enough, "Egg Replacer" stands in reasonably well in most recipes. The best cookie and the best
brownie I've ever eaten have both been vegan, and there are any
number of vegan cookbooks that offer up sensational egg-free
baked desserts.

There is even a great vegan omelet I can recommend. Su-
san Voisin at FatFreeVegan.com has posted a "Vegan Omelet for
One" recipe[1]. If an omelet seems too fancy, try a tofu scramble:
an egg-like meal so simple it hardly requires a formal recipe. Just
sauté some sliced onions, garlic, and peppers, add some mashed
firm tofu, and then stir in some nutritional yeast and tamari
before serving.

Gaining More than Losing

One of this book's themes is that a successful transition to being
vegan requires that you focus on adding foods to your diet, rather
than putting emphasis on subtracting foods. Undoubtedly, if
you're a big fan of T-bone steaks or sunny side up eggs, a vegan
diet means doing without a convincing replacement. But as we've
seen in this chapter, most other animal products are easily and
gracefully replaced by a variety of vegan items. In terms of the
pleasure you take from eating, the foods you'll discover should
more than make up for the foods you subtract.

---

[1]http://tinyurl.com/2hgapj

Chapter 20

Outfitting Your Kitchen

When I became vegan in the late 1980s, veggie-friendly restaurants were so scarce, and vegan convenience foods so few, that you might starve if you didn't learn how to cook. Today, the situation isn't nearly so bleak, but a little cooking ability still goes a long way. So the next few chapters will help you get more comfortable in the kitchen.

You can't start cooking until you've outfitted your kitchen with the basics. So in this chapter I will cover essential items for the kitchen.

To begin, you of course need cookware. Get a largish kettle and a smallish pot. You'll use these for everything from making rice to reheating yesterday's soup. You don't need to spend much money on these, since the cheapest enamel-coated metal pots are a terrific choice. You'll also need a pan or two for sautéing vegetables and for stir-fries. Here, I recommend getting a large stainless steel skillet; one of these will last for decades, and they make cooking a pleasure. If you can afford one, buy a wok as well—they are incomparable for making Chinese-style stir-fry dishes. Finally, you'll need at least one baking sheet.

For your pots, pans, and baking sheets, I recommend avoiding nonstick surfaces, as they contain some nasty chemicals. Plus, even with proper care, nonstick cookware survives only a few years of regular use. By contrast, you'll find that cast iron, stainless steel, and enamel-coated cookware is nearly indestructible.

Buy some wooden spoons, and also a spatula or two, for mixing soups, removing items from baking sheets, and for stir-frying vegetables.

You'll also need kitchen knives and at least one cutting board. Get a quality three to five piece knife set—kitchen knives are always much cheaper when purchased in a set. Chicago Cutlery is a great mid-priced brand. Whatever you do, don't buy cheap kitchen knives; they dull quickly and will turn your cooking experiences into an unnecessary hassle. Also, buy the largest white polypropylene cutting board you can find. Wooden cutting boards look nice, but they pick up odors and are harder to keep clean.

Here are a few final accessories you'll need. Buy a chrome four-sided cheese grater—you'll use it all the time for grating vegetables for salads. You'll need a vegetable peeler plus some measuring cups and spoons. You should also get a set of mixing bowls—inexpensive ones work fine. A citrus juicer is another essential accessory: I prefer the cheap two-piece models featuring a plastic reamer screwed onto a glass jar.

With these accessories out of the way, let's now move on to what I regard as the three kitchen appliances you can't live without: a blender, a two slot toaster, and a George Foreman grill. If you go cheap, you can get all this for $50 or so. Even the cheapest blenders work well; I prefer glass blender pitchers to plastic. Pretty much all blenders manufactured today allow you to unscrew the pitcher's bottom to clean the propeller—make sure yours does.

Toasters aren't worth spending much money on since even the cheapest ones work admirably. If you're a bagel-eater, buy a toaster with self-adjusting slots. Slot toasters make toast faster than toaster ovens, and the toast comes out better too. I use mine all the time.

George Foreman grills are indispensable for grilling veggies, especially broccoli, cauliflower, and peppers. You would think a George Foreman grill would be the ultimate way to cook veggieburgers, but I prefer to pan fry them in a bit of oil—sadly, veggieburgers don't contain enough fat to come out well when cooked in an electric grill.

Now let's cover a few more appliances that, while not quite mandatory, can further improve your quality of life.

If you like beans, you *must* own a pressure cooker—you'll be able to cook dried beans from scratch in a small fraction of the time it would take to prepare them in a kettle. These devices also save a lot of energy as your food requires much less time to cook. If you enjoy artichokes, you'll find that pressure cookers also make wonderful steamers.

On the other end of the stovetop cooking spectrum, but comparably useful, is a slow-cooker—which most people refer to using the trademarked name of Crock-Pot. Whatever you call these devices, slow-cookers offer an amazing way to prepare soups. You throw in a bunch of veggies and spices and come back hours later to piping-hot, perfectly cooked soup. Some people start their slow-cookers in the morning and drive off to work, but I think that's insane. I would never leave a $20 electrical appliance operating unattended, since it's a house fire waiting to happen. But if you're going to be home all day, nothing beats a slow-cooker. It takes only a few minutes to chop your veggies for a big pot of soup. I don't have a favorite brand of slow-cooker but I do recommend you spend a few extra dollars to get one that features removable stoneware, which makes cleanup a breeze.

My bread machine has paid for itself many times over, since I can make a small loaf of organic bread for less than fifty cents. I've got a West Bend Just-for-Dinner bread machine that kneads and then bakes a loaf about the size of a softball—perfect for two people—in 45 minutes flat. Most bread machines come with recipes that call for dairy products, but you can safely substitute vegan margarine in place of butter. In bread machine recipes that call for cow's milk, I've successfully used water or unsweetened soymilk instead.

If you are passionate about cooking, or you regularly cook for large groups, you should buy a food processor. Cuisinart offers a unit (model BFP-10CH) that includes both a blender pitcher and a food processor bowl, so this is nice a way to purchase an upscale food processor and a blender, while saving space and money at the same time.

If you're one of those people who has fits getting rice to turn out right, you will love owning a rice cooker. You just measure out your rice and water, turn it on, and it'll make perfect rice every time. I recommend avoiding rice cookers with aluminum pots just to be on the safe side, as the toxicity of aluminum cookware is still in dispute.

Finally, let's take a quick look at juicers. Juicers are one of those things people buy with great intentions but frequently never use. There are two kinds of home juicers: centrifugal and masticating. Centrifugal juicers have cheaper and smaller motors and you can get one of well under $100. The best known masticating juicer, made by Champion, costs over $200 and will last forever. Masticating juicers make a better grade of juice because they thoroughly tear up the cells of whatever fruit or vegetable you're using. Also, masticating juicers can be much easier to clean than centrifugal juicers. The one disadvantage of masticating juicers is that they are surprisingly heavy. I wouldn't buy a Champion unless I had enough kitchen countertop space to leave it there permanently.

If you're planning to make a lot of juice, I suggest investing in a Champion. You might want to check Craigslist.org or the bulletin board at your local natural foods store to see if you can find a used one. Owing to the famous durability of Champions, used should be as good as new, and I wouldn't spend more than

$70 on a used Champion.

So that's it. Pick up the items mentioned in this chapter and you'll have the kitchen equipment you need for 99 percent of the recipes you see in cookbooks. Remember, you want being vegan to be as easy as possible, so be sure to purchase any kitchen items you're confident that you'll regularly use.

Chapter 21

Core Foods: Smoothies & Sandwiches

Although cookbooks can teach you a lot about cooking, it's a vastly better use of your time to learn how to make core foods than it is to learn specific recipes. What are core foods? They are foods that can form the core of your diet because they satisfy four criteria:

- They are quick and easy to make, since you obviously don't want your diet to be heavily based on fussy foods that take forever to prepare.

- Any one core food can be prepared in numerous ways, so it doesn't seem like you're eating the exact same food every single day.

- They are healthful. It's OK to eat the occasional chocolate bar or bag of potato chips, but the foods that form the core of your diet had better be good for you and loaded with nutrients.

- This final quality should be common sense: your core foods need to be so delicious that you'll *want* to eat them every day.

In this chapter, we'll cover two core foods that I think you'll love: fruit smoothies and sandwiches. Over the course of this chapter, we'll see that these two foods are easy to make, taste great, are highly nutritious, and can be prepared from different ingredients every time.

Smoothies

Smoothies may be the easiest food you'll ever make—even if you don't know how to boil water you can make a smoothie. The whole process takes thirty seconds, with cleanup being almost as quick. You start with some sort of vegan milk: soymilk, almond milk, rice milk, hempseed milk, whatever. Put a cup or two of your vegan milk in a blender and then drop in a handful of frozen fruit, and give it a whirl until everything is thoroughly blended.

One virtue of smoothies is they're a perfect place to toss in a tablespoon or two of ground flax seeds, so you can get your full day's worth of Omega 3s, plus a nice serving of fruit, just as you're starting up your day.

The best part about smoothies is that you can mix up your fruits from one day to the next. You can buy numerous varieties of bagged frozen fruit at any supermarket or natural foods store.

As delicious as fruit smoothies are, they taste even better when you've picked and prepared the fruit yourself. One of my favorite summertime activities is to visit a you-pick orchard or berry farm, and spend a couple hours picking my favorite fruits. When I get home, I'll wash and then cut up the fruit, then freeze everything in single layers on baking sheets until all my fruit is rock-hard. At that point I transfer the fruit to gallon-sized freezer bags for storage in my freezer. The tray-based preparation technique I just described is called IQF (Individually Quick Freezing), and it ensures that the fruit in your freezer bag doesn't freeze together into an unappetizing icy brick. I also use this IQF technique for freezing peeled and sliced bananas.

You can further increase your smoothie variety by blending two or more fruits at once. Today you might prepare a blueberry-strawberry smoothie and tomorrow you might enjoy a smoothie made from apricots and blackberries.

Sandwiches

Let's now move on to this chapter's other core food: sandwiches. While you can concoct a wide assortment of smoothies, the variety of sandwiches you can create is near-infinite.

First, the bread. If you've got a bread machine, you can continually change up the variety of breads you make: whole wheat, rye, raisin, multigrain, and so forth. Many bread machine recipes nicely accommodate the addition of a tablespoon of ground flax, which helps boost your intake of Omega 3s. Whatever bread you select, whole grain varieties are the most nutritious.

You can keep things interesting by occasionally making your sandwich from a bagel instead of sliced bread. Also, anything you can put in a sandwich could just as easily go into a tortilla-based wrap. My favorite brand of tortilla is made by Alvarado Street Bakery. They make small and large whole grain tortillas from sprouted organic wheat. These tortillas are frozen and distributed to natural food stores across the United States. I often heat these tortillas for a few seconds on each side in a skillet over low heat. This not only provides some welcome warmth, it also softens up the tortilla so it'll roll into a wrap without breaking.

Let's now look at possible sandwich fillings. Perhaps the most popular sandwich in America is the old standby, peanut butter and jelly. As I mentioned in a previous chapter, jams and preserves are tastier and more nutritious than jelly. Additionally, many people don't realize that peanut butter is only the beginning of their nut butter options. You can choose all sorts of other nut butters that are widely sold at natural food stores. Almond butter is great, I adore cashew butter and macadamia butter, and pistachio butter is difficult to find but is my favorite option of all.

There are plenty of other great sandwich fillings. Hummus is fantastic on a sandwich along with some thinly-sliced tomato and either sprouts or finely-chopped parsley. You might want to add some sliced olives and a few drops of hot sauce as well. And remember that there are innumerable varieties of hummus—many vegan cookbooks feature especially creative varieties.

Vegan sliced meats can be found at any natural foods store. Sliced seitan can be great as well. Smoked, grilled, or baked tofu, cut into thin slices, is a terrific sandwich filling. One of my mother's favorite foods is a BLT made with a vegan product called Smart Bacon.

Every once in a while I get a craving for a grilled cheese sandwich. I'll grate or thinly slice some vegan cheese, and then, before grilling, I'll butter the bread with vegan margarine.

When you add up all the varieties of bread, bagels, tortillas, fillings, veggies, and spreads that could possibly go into a sandwich, you start to see that the possibilities are nearly limitless.

As nutritious as smoothies and sandwiches are, these foods won't be adding many vegetables to your diet. In order to boost our consumption of healthy vegetables, we'll next look at three more core foods: salads, stir-fries, and grilled veggies.

Chapter **22**

More Core Foods: Salads, Stir-Fries, & Grilled Veggies

In this chapter, we'll look at how to create terrific salads, stir-fries, and grilled veggies. Each of these foods deserves to be a regular part of your diet—they are super healthful, delicious, and can be prepared in countless ways.

Salads

Salads are one of the easiest foods you could ever prepare, but I've nevertheless got a few pieces of advice that will make your salads far more appealing. First, if you eat any salads at all, you absolutely and positively need to buy a salad spinner. Without a salad spinner, your greens never get quite dry. And, if they're even slightly wet, your dressing will run right off, like water hitting a raincoat—which is only to be expected given that oil and water don't mix. When you buy your salad spinner, make sure it's a big one. As we're about to see, even if you live alone, it

121

makes sense to prepare a lot of salad at once.

The problem with salads is that even though they're easy to prepare, it's a lot of work to make just one salad. By the time you select, wash, and cut up your veggies you've invested a fair amount of time for not a lot of food. And when you're hungry, who really wants to go through all that hassle? It's a lot easier to eat convenience food.

So here's an idea that will get you eating tons more salad: go to any department store and buy five or six plastic storage containers that each hold a large serving of salad. Or, you can buy containers large enough to hold two servings if you typically dine with your partner. You can then make a full week's worth of salad at one time, with each salad ready-to-eat in its own container. Anytime you're hungry you'll know that you've got freshly-made salad in the refrigerator just waiting to be pulled out. Salads stored in these containers are also perfect for bringing to work.

If possible, put the salad on a plate before eating since these plastic containers can be tough to get clean if they come in contact with oily salad dressings. And never store salad with dressing already applied—doing so will wilt your greens within hours.

Now let's look at salad ingredients. Any kind of lettuce, spinach, or chard makes a great base. Dandelion greens deserve to be widely used in salads since they're a delicious choice. But if you hate lettuce or greens, then skip them, and just make your salad from chopped veggies. As long as a vegetable can be eaten raw, it can go into your salad. Try to select as many differently colored vegetables as possible, as that produces a more beautiful salad, and a greater variety of distinct flavors. I especially like purple cabbage, grated carrots, and thinly-sliced sweet peppers.

You can of course use any vegan bottled dressing, but I generally don't recommend bottled dressings because they're overpriced and often mediocre. About the only bottled dressing I think is truly tasty is Annie's Goddess Dressing. Happily, Annie's is the one dressing that can be purchased inexpensively: you can buy food-service sized one liter bottles from Amazon.com for a very reasonable price.

An even better option is to make your own dressing, and it's amazingly easy. My favorite homemade dressing is also the simplest. Just take some tahini, and stir in some lemon juice, minced garlic, and salt. Then mix in water until you've attained a creamy texture. I never get tired of tahini dressing, but if you do, you'll have one more reason to buy a copy of Robin Robertson's *Vegan Planet*—you may remember me raving about this cookbook in Chapter 4. The salad section of *Vegan Planet* contains recipes for more than thirty different dressings.

Finally, don't even think about serving that salad without some nice toppings. Here are some great ones: sliced olives, chopped nuts, tamari roasted sunflower seeds, chopped basil, thin slices of baked marinated tofu, finely chopped parsley, vegan croutons, and sprouts. Americans don't eat much salad because they don't eat much *good* salad. Once you start making salads like this it's easy for your salad-eating to become a daily habit.

Stir-Fries

Nearly all vegetables suitable for salads, lettuce obviously excepted, are also great in stir-fries. To make a stir-fry, you wash your veggies, peel them if necessary, and then cut them into bite-sized pieces. Next, you'll sauté the veggies at a temperature that's not quite hot enough to scorch the oil. You want to keep your veggies constantly moving, hence the name stir-fry, so that they are nicely seared by the heat but not burned.

A wok is the ideal stir-fry pan, but you can also use a large skillet. Use an oil like coconut oil or high oleic safflower oil that can stand up to high temperatures.

You should add the coarse, heavy veggies first, like yams, eggplant, potatoes, carrots or winter squash. You'll need to cut these sorts of veggies pretty thinly or they won't cook through. After a few minutes of stir-frying, add in some lighter veggies like zucchini, broccoli, cauliflower, or sliced peppers. Make sure you peel your broccoli or cauliflower before adding because otherwise the thick skins will prevent the stalks from getting adequately cooked. Keep stir-frying a few more minutes, and after everything is almost cooked add some chopped leafy greens. Just before serving, you might throw in some minced garlic and ginger and allow it to sizzle just a bit before stirring into the mix. I also love to stir in some chopped basil or cilantro at the very end. Other times, I'll add a peanut or coconut sauce, or perhaps some tamari or hot sauce.

The best way to learn how to cook stir-fries is to watch someone who's done it for a while. It's easy once you get the hang of it. Like salads, stir-fries are a fantastic core food since it takes no effort to change up the veggies you use from one day to the next. Also, like salads, try to use as many differently colored veggies as possible for optimum taste, appearance, and nutrition.

You can serve stir-fries over rice, millet, quinoa—just about any grain you like. I'll often serve mine without a grain just to get a big easy-to-digest dose of veggies.

There's an easy way to rapidly improve your stir-fry skills: when you eat your stir-fry, taste each separate vegetable individually and ask yourself if it's perfectly cooked. If you've undercooked your sweet potatoes or overcooked your broccoli, you'll know better next time. By taking the time to judge how each veggie in your stir-fry turned out, you'll quickly become a stir-fry master.

Grilled Vegetables

I've already raved in this book about my George Foreman grill, which is probably a surprise recommendation given that this product is mainly associated with hamburgers. It's definitely one of my top three kitchen appliances, and the cheapest model can be had for only about $20.

To me, there's no better way to cook broccoli and cauliflower than in a George Foreman. The combination of grilling and steaming that takes place in a George Foreman-style grill makes it the perfect way to cook these veggies. As with stir-frying, you'll want to remove the skins from all stalks. I'll usually rotate each piece a quarter turn after five minutes or so, to ensure the veggies are uniformly seared. When your veggies are grilled to the degree you want, put them in a bowl and spoon on a little Earth Balance margarine, which will quickly melt.

You can have success grilling other veggies as well, such as sliced onions, eggplant, and summer squash. These vegetables are especially good when marinated in a tamari-based seasoned sauce prior to grilling. Sweet peppers are also fantastic when grilled but they're also the one veggie that tends to dirty up a George Foreman.

***

When you consider all the veggies you can eat through salads, stir-fries, and grilling, you'll appreciate how these three core foods put you in a position to dramatically increase the variety of healthful vegetables in your diet.

We've covered food, food, and more food over the course of this book. We've looked at restaurant food, grocery shopping, convenience foods, food preparation, you name it. After all this eating, we need something to wash it down. So I'll devote our next chapter to everything liquid, from water to soymilk to booze.

Chapter 23

Beverages

One of the ironies of veganism is that many people won't try it for fear their diets would become too limited, and yet when you meet most long-term vegans you quickly realize that their diets are way more varied, delicious, and healthful than a typical omnivore's. Perhaps that's only to be expected because the act of becoming vegan requires that you start paying more attention to food—and this extra attention quickly pays big dividends.

Just as it's worthwhile to become a minor authority on food, there are things you can learn about beverages that will deliver big payoffs.

Water

Noted alcoholic W.C. Fields once said, "Say anything that you like about me except that I drink water."

Like W.C. Fields, most Americans have a curious and counterproductive relationship with water. We know the stuff coming out of the tap often tastes nasty, so many people respond by paying exorbitant prices for bottled water. Obviously, we should all be drinking the purest water we can get. But there's no reason why this water must come at great expense, or that it needs to waste large amounts of plastic.

I think the best way to get water is through a reverse osmosis system. In my opinion, carbon-based filters just aren't effective enough at removing contaminants and delivering optimum taste.

A reverse osmosis filter contains a special kind of membrane that permits almost nothing but water molecules to go through. These systems include pre-filtering components so that the membrane doesn't immediately get clogged. Reverse osmosis filtered water is about as pure as water can be; it's nearly as pure as distilled—but much cheaper and much less wasteful of energy. It tastes as good as the best spring water.

You've got three options for obtaining reverse osmosis water: you can purchase the water from stores, you can install a unit in your home, or you can buy a portable unit. Let's look at each of these options.

Many supermarkets and natural food stores have machines that dispense reverse osmosis water into jugs that you bring to refill, at a cost of 25 to 50 cents a gallon. In warmer climates these machines are often located outside in front of supermarkets and drug stores. Check the information printed on the machine to be sure the system includes a reverse osmosis filter. The cost of buying water from a machine is dirt cheap compared to bottled water, but it's still much more expensive than owning a reverse osmosis unit, where the cost works out to only pennies a gallon. Plus, buying your own reverse osmosis system means you'll have one less regular errand to make, and you won't have to be lugging water jugs in and out of your house.

If you own your home, you can buy an under-the-sink reverse osmosis unit. These units used to cost close to $500, but now you can get a good one for under $150. A plumber should need about two hours to install your unit, so you're probably looking at another $250 or so for labor. After that, your only expense will be changing the filters, which you can do yourself, and which should only cost another $50 a year, or possibly $100 if you've got a large and thirsty family.

Finally, even if you're renting, you're not out of luck. You can purchase a countertop reverse osmosis unit that hooks up to your kitchen faucet. You might have some trouble if your faucet is older or has a non-standard design, but if you've got a modern kitchen sink setup, a countertop unit can be a fantastic choice. And since these units have a simpler design than under-the-sink models, they're really cheap: about $100. Whether countertop or under-the-sink, you can buy reverse osmosis units at any home improvement center, from Amazon.com, or through eBay.

My only warning about reverse osmosis systems is that these units may not be able to handle well-water. Some well-water is too hard for a reverse osmosis unit to handle, and many well pumps don't deliver adequate water pressure to drive a reverse osmosis unit. But if your house gets city water you should be in great shape.

Vegan Milks

Now that we've gotten water out of the way, let's move on to non-dairy milks, You can get these made from soy, rice, almonds, and even hempseeds. They're all pretty good. Rice milk is a little too thin for my taste, and it's not as nutritious as other vegan milks. You might think think hempseed milk would taste nasty, but it's surprisingly delicious, and it also packs Omega 3s, which the others don't.

Soymilk has been around for centuries, and you can buy traditional soymilk in gallon jugs at any Asian grocery. Don't. The traditional stuff is unsweetened and has a weird taste. It turns out that when you boil down soybeans to make soymilk, the soy protein denatures, which produces a bizarre flavor. All the national brands use some sort of high-tech method to get rid of this denatured protein, and taste much better as a result. I've got some Asian friends who grew up drinking the traditional stuff and who therefore think it tastes fine. But for everyone else, I strongly recommend sticking with the national brands.

By the way, the dairy interests hate it when companies use the word milk in conjunction with a vegan product. They've even tried to make doing so illegal. So I go out of my way to use the word milk at every opportunity when talking about these vegan beverages and I encourage you to do the same.

Whether you buy soy, almond, rice, or hempseed milk, these products are usually available in plain, chocolate, and vanilla flavors. Try to find a brand that's fortified with Vitamin B_{12}, as it's always good to take in a little extra B_{12} here and there in addition to your daily supplement. You *are* taking B_{12} in your daily multivitamin, plus a sublingual B_{12} tablet a couple times a week, aren't you?

I've got one final tip regarding soymilk. If you've got a Costco membership, you can buy a three-pack of half-gallon containers for about the same price as two half-gallons would cost anywhere else. The product, sold under Costco's Kirkwood label, is organic and there's no better soymilk on the market. I always favor refrigerated soymilk in paper milk cartons over the stuff in aseptic juice boxes, as it's far less wasteful of resources.

Booze

Now let's move on to some info for everyone who is 21 and over, or who has a good fake ID. It's time for me to offer a vegan take on beer, wine, and distilled spirits.

The first thing you need to know is that many beers and wines are made with tiny amounts of animal ingredients. Note that I wrote, "made with," and not, "contain." Here's the deal with my choice of words. When you make beer or wine you've got a fermenting liquid in which tiny grain pieces or grape particles are floating around. You can let the mixture stand for a week or so and everything will settle to the bottom, and you could then decant the liquid free of any insoluble particles. But that means letting your product occupy your fermentation vat for extra time, and many winemakers and beer brewers want to hurry things along. So they'll often throw in some fish gelatin, which is called isinglass, or they'll add some egg whites to the mix. This non-vegan nastiness will clump up with all the undissolved stuff in the vat, at which point everything—fish or egg gunk and sediments alike—can easily be strained out of the mix using a fine screen.

So there are two things to keep in mind. Number one is that there's no fish gelatin or animal products to speak of that remain in the wine or beer you drink, since it's all filtered off. And number two, the amount of fish gel or egg whites used is tiny, and fish gel is a byproduct of the fishing industry that provides them with next to nothing in the way of profits. Also, some people are allergic to even minute amounts of egg whites, so winemakers are under constant pressure to discontinue their use of egg products.

Still, I admit, it's a gross out that the stuff may be used in the first place. It's really just a way for beer and winemakers to boost output by dedicating their vats solely to fermenting. Luckily, most brewers and many winemakers produce a totally vegan product, and it's easy to find out which brands are vegan. You can just visit my buddy Jason's site, barnivore.com, to check out his comprehensive vegan beer and wine lists. Additionally, Appendix C features a short selection of the most popular vegan beers.

Now, I admit, the thought of looking up the vegan status of beers and wines may drive you to drink the hard stuff. But that's cool, because nearly every brand of distilled spirit is vegan. To paraphrase George Thorogood, our friends Jimmy Beam, Jack Daniels, Johnnie Walker, and even our dear Old Grand-Dad are vegan. Oddly enough, you can even drink all the Wild Turkey you want and not a single bird will be harmed, only your liver. In fact, as long as you're not drinking some sort of floofy sweet creamy liqueur, which is for sissies anyway, any rotgut you're imbibing is vegan-friendly.

This chapter's coverage of beer and wine has forced me onto the subject of hidden animal ingredients, a topic that unfortunately extends far beyond alcoholic beverages. So in the next chapter we'll look much more closely at hidden animal ingredients, and I'll give you the inside scoop.

Chapter 24

Animal Ingredients

Would you like to eliminate something like 97 percent of your consumption of animal products? Simple: just stop eating foods that contain ingredients that are clearly derived from meat, milk, and eggs. Want to go further? Again, it's simple: avoid products containing leather, wool, or silk. Now you've probably eliminated 99.8 percent of your animal product consumption.

All of this is pretty easy. But here's the bummer: once you've taken these steps, the law of diminishing returns kicks in and eradicating that final trace of animal products from your life is next to impossible. Luckily, as we'll see in this chapter, there's really no point in aspiring to total vegan purity. Nobody is absolutely, positively vegan, and there are frankly far more meaningful and productive ways to spend your time than obsessing about reaching an indisputable 100 percent vegan status.

The reason that animal products are hard to completely avoid is that they can show up almost anywhere, and this is because animal agriculture generates tremendous quantities of byproducts. The United States alone raises and slaughters well over 10 billion animals each year. Whether we're talking cattle or pigs or chickens, well over 30 percent of their weight is essentially unwanted—consisting of blood, skin, bone, excess fat, organ flesh, and so forth. While it's true that leather generates relatively high value, most of the remaining byproducts are almost, but not completely, worthless.

So we're talking about millions and millions of tons of waste products generated by slaughterhouses each year in the United States. What do they do with all this stuff? They extract this material into nasty scab-like piles, and everything that doesn't go into pet food is processed into various food and industrial chemicals. Let's now look at where these chemicals end up.

If you've ever spent time reading food labels, you know that processed food often includes all sorts of unpronounceable chemicals. Now, obviously, the average person has no way to figure out if a given food chemical comes from an animal, vegetable, or mineral. But somebody with a background in chemistry would certainly know, right? Wrong. That's because nearly every substance that food companies source from a slaughterhouse is derived from either protein or fat. And here things get confusing, because, just like slaughterhouse byproducts, the plant kingdom is filled with proteins and fats as well. So, most of the time, all you can know about a given food ingredient bearing a chemical name is that it *might* be derived from animal sources.

As a consequence, in most cases there is really no way to figure out a given chemical's vegan status, because sometimes it's sourced from slaughterhouse byproducts, while other times that very same chemical will be sourced from plant-based ingredients. Ten years ago there was a very popular book on the subject, which gave vegans the impression that they could just look up a given food ingredient and gain some certainty over where it came from. But as we've just seen, there's really no way to reliably compile a comprehensive list. A high percentage of food chemicals deserve "maybe" status, which is completely unhelpful.

If you sincerely want to keep any trace of animal ingredients from showing up in your food, the solution is easy: don't focus on the origin of obscure ingredients, just eat real food—fruits, veggies, grains, rice, beans, nuts, and so forth. And don't buy any processed crap that contains ingredients you can't pronounce. Easy enough, huh?

Having said that, it's still desirable to learn about the animal ingredients that are most likely to show up in processed food. Many of these have innocent-sounding names that don't betray their animal origin. Here's a quick run through of words to look out for:

- Carmine or anything that sounds like it is a red food coloring made from ground-up beetles. Yeah, I know. Totally disgusting.

- Casein and similar-sounding substances are milk proteins.

- Collagen, glycerine, and keratin are all rendered slaughterhouse ingredients.

- Gelatin is derived from the skins or bones of animals.

- Glycerine, lactic acid, mono or diglycerides, and stearic acid can be produced from slaughterhouse fat, but they could also be vegan.

- Lactose is a sugar extracted from milk.

- Lard and tallow are both are fancy names for animal fat.

- Whey is a milk-based byproduct of cheese making.

Obviously, this short collection of items only scratches the surface of all the animal products out there. But I've at least given you the most common ones to keep in mind and watch out for.

While it's fairly easy to banish animal ingredients from your food just by avoiding processed stuff, you should be aware that it's next to impossible to eradicate all traces of animal products from your life. Consider, for example, a bicycle, the epitome of green living—the steel in its frame might have been lubricated at the steel mill using animal fat, and the rubber in its tires was probably vulcanized with tallow.

Since traces of animal products are widely used in all sorts of factory production, I've seen meat producers argue that, if it weren't for animal agriculture, commerce would grind to a halt. This is probably the most unintelligent argument ever made by anyone on any subject. Nearly all the animal products used by industry are derived from fats or proteins, and the only reason these substances are sourced from animal rather than plant ingredients is so producers can save a few pennies.

I hope I've successfully made the argument that there's really no way to remove all traces of animal products from your lifestyle, and that focusing on microscopic quantities of animal products is counterproductive. If you're vegan and you make a point of avoiding the places where animal products show up in quantity in manufactured goods—principly clothing, shoes, furniture, and car seats, you're really doing everything you could be possibly expected to do.

So once you've stopped eating animal-based foods, and you're not buying things like leather sofas and wool or silk-based clothing, there's just one more set of products that is worth your attention: cosmetics and personal care items are the final place that animal products show up in significant quantity. For instance, a typical bar of soap can be made almost entirely of animal fat. It's therefore sensible to ensure that that the soaps, detergents, shampoos, and conditioners you buy are are vegetable-based. Ditto for laundry and dish detergent. It's easy to find vegetable-based versions of all these products online or at your local natural food store. And obviously, it's also worthwhile to make sure that these items aren't tested on animals: personal care products and household cleaners usually carry a prominent label if they were formulated without animal tests.

As we've seen, it's easy to banish the major and minor sources of animal products from of your life. And happily, what minuscule traces of animal ingredients remain won't deliver measurable profit to animal agribusiness.

After you've done the things recommended in this chapter, I hope you won't let a few molecules of animal fat in your bicycle tires be a concern. As we'll see in this book's final chapter, it's infinitely more productive to devote your attention to getting involved in outreach and activism.

Chapter 25

Friends & Family

In this chapter, we're going to consider the influence your dietary choices may have on your friends and family. It's all too easy, especially as a new vegan, to come off as a freak to the people closest to you. So in this chapter we will look at how to present your eating habits in the most favorable light.

If possible, you should avoid talking about vegan topics when you're still new to the lifestyle, because early on you probably won't yet be knowledgeable enough to discuss the issues convincingly. And if you present the issues badly the first time, you often don't get a second chance. So before you talk to others about how and why to be vegan, it makes sense to read a few books on the subject. The more informed you are, the more effectively you'll be able to talk about your diet—whether your audience is your parents, your spouse, your co-workers, or your classmates.

Books like Tom Regan's *Empty Cages* and Singer and Mason's *The Ethics of What We Eat* offer a solid background on how to speak about the ethical issues surrounding diet. And my own book *Meat Market* offers a more detailed and research-heavy overview of animal agribusiness than what I offered in the first two chapters of this book.

Because so many people are more concerned with health than

with ethics, it also makes sense to read some health-oriented vegan books. *Becoming Vegan* by Davis and Melina is a good choice. And, since many people have heart disease in their family, Caldwell Esselstyn's *Prevent and Reverse Heart Disease* is another important book to read. Fitness is another hot topic for vegans, and people concerned with athletic performance will find Brendan Brazier's *The Thrive Diet* to be worthwhile.

Finally, as I mentioned earlier in this book, I strongly recommend you read everything at Jack Norris' VeganHealth.org site. The stuff there is rock solid in terms of credibility, and this collection of articles offers a thorough overview of all issues related to vegan nutrition.

After you've read all this material, you'll know more about food than 99 percent of Americans. And as a result, you'll be able to discuss the issues surrounding vegan food choices with a level of expertise that will surprise and impress the people in your life. When it comes to winning people over to thinking favorably of vegan eating, there's just no substitute to becoming well-versed in all of the primary ethical and health issues connected to diet. Acquiring this breadth of knowledge will make your discussions with family, friends, and co-workers smoother, easier, and vastly more productive.

Everything I just said about reading several books goes double if you're still living with your parents, and it goes triple if you're under age fifteen. I became vegetarian when I was nineteen, and when I broke the news to my mother, you would think from her reaction that I had just announced my intention to become a professional skydiver. Happily, in short order I was able to convince her that I was taking my nutrition seriously and therefore wouldn't get myself in any trouble.

For most kids who become vegan, their parents' worries stem from knowing little about nutrition, and wrongfully believing that veganism is an inadequate diet that will lead to stunted growth and health problems. So if you're a child or adolescent, it may be worthwhile to trot out the American Dietetic Association's position paper on vegetarian diets. This document concludes that a well-planned vegan diet is appropriate for every stage of life, including pregnancy, infancy, adolescence, and old age. You can find a supposedly non-printable PDF version of this paper on the web.[1]

To the extent that you can get your parents to read books about vegan diets, so much the better. If that's something they won't go for, you can at least get ahold of some Vegan Outreach brochures. These are short, full of photos, and highly informative. Always be sure that any literature you offer speaks to your recipient's interests. If your mother is a big animal lover, it makes sense to give her literature that talks about factory farming. If your dad doesn't care much about animals, but has heart disease on both sides of his family, it would be appropriate to get a Caldwell Esselstyn book into his hands.

No matter how receptive your parents are, living at home can still lead to problems, especially at first. I spent my sophomore year of college living at my parents' house, and my mother did most of the grocery shopping. One day she came home with a half dozen cans of vegetable soup. But when I checked the label I saw these soups contained chicken stock. No problem. I just telephoned the vegan police and they came right over, arrested my mother, and took her to a vegan re-education camp. I have no idea of what she experienced at the camp, but I must say that after she returned, she was always super vigilant when it came to thoroughly reading the labels of anything she bought for me.

In all seriousness, my parents have become quite understanding and supportive of my vegan diet. And while they haven't gone vegan, my mother often has vegan days. The amount of animal products they eat today is substantially less than it used to be.

---

[1]They keep moving this darned thing around. With luck, you can still find it here: http://www.eatright.org/ada/files/vegnp.pdf

Many of the ideas I've just expressed about dealing with parents apply similarly to romantic relationships. It's important to realize that if you've been with your partner for a while and have just become vegan, he or she is likely to feel somewhat threatened by or resentful over your change of diet—something along the lines of: "Hey, I never signed up for this."

Here, however, you'll have more leverage than a teenager has with his or her parents. Any relationship ought to be based on having concern for the interests and values of your partner, so, if you've just become vegan, it's your job to clearly express why it's important to you. As I mentioned at the start of this chapter, it's wise to defer these conversations until after you've had a chance to read a few books, so that you can introduce the subject in an informed and convincing manner.

It's hard to accurately predict how your partner will respond. Some partners—most often men—view the entire veggie concept with hostility and distrust. They'll actually go out of their way to be unaccommodating. To me, hostile reactions like this, particularly if they accompany ridicule, have no place in a relationship. If you find yourself in this sort of situation, the issues surrounding diet are likely to be the least of your relationship's concerns. You've got to wonder about the overall health of the relationship, and unless kids are in the picture I'd recommend putting some thought into whether to ditch the jerk.

Many partners, however, are simply fantastic. They'll realize that your change of diet is greatly important to you, and take it upon themselves to do the requisite reading. Often, after exploring the subject, they'll jump right on board and become vegan too. If this is the reaction you get, marry this person.

And finally, there are partners who'll bend halfway. They might be willing to go veggie or even vegan in the house, and when you eat out together they'll make a point of not ordering the ribs in front of you. One vegan I know is married to a man who is mostly vegan apart from one night a week when he dines omnivorously with friends at a restaurant.

Let's finish off this chapter by considering how to create the most productive impression among your friends concerning your food choices. The most important thing I can tell you is to avoid putting yourself at the center of this topic. It's not about you being vegan. It's about the delicious food you're eating, it's about heaping scorn upon a corrupt and brutal factory farming industry, and it's about making the healthiest possible food choices.

As with every other interaction we have, we influence people most when we listen closely rather than talk. By discovering which areas of interest are of greatest concern to the people in your life, you can figure out exactly what sorts of information each person would be most responsive to.

There are some other tricks you'll learn along the way. Never agree to eat out with friends if it means that you'll be at a place where your meal will look meager or unappetizing compared to your companions' omnivorous choices. If you love to cook and are great at it, invite your friends over for a special meal based on a sensational recipe you've already mastered. See, at every turn you're presenting your food choices as fun, delicious, healthful, and carefully thought out.

It's not like all your friends are likely to go vegan overnight, but when you've read deeply into the literature and can present your diet in a positive manner you can expect to have a tremendous influence among the people in your circle. Rather than being looked at as freakish for your food choices, the decisions you've made about diet will instead seem admirable and worthy of emulation.

If you present things correctly, it's amazing the influence you'll have. Over the years, many of the people closest to me have become vegan. And those who have not gone vegan have nevertheless made substantial changes to how they eat. I don't think there's a single person left in my life who would set foot inside a McDonald's or KFC. And all of this has occurred without any confrontation, any proselytizing, or any hard feelings.

As we've seen, if you become well-versed on the subject of vegan eating and learn to talk about it effectively, you're likely to become a positive and powerful influence on how your friends and loved ones eat.

Chapter **26**

Staying Motivated

We've now covered everything you need to know in order to transition to a vegan diet. Once you've learned the basics, going vegan is mainly about being properly motivated. Let's quickly review the main things you can do to stay motivated:

- Read vegan-oriented books. You'll learn things that will make your transition easier, and make you more excited to be vegan.

- Try new vegan foods every day. Every new food you discover pushes you closer to becoming a lifelong vegan.

- Spend time learning to prepare vegan foods, especially the core foods covered in Chapters 21 and 22.

- Regularly dine out at veggie-friendly restaurants.

- Attend local vegan Meetup.com events, and get active with your local vegetarian and animal protection groups.

- Subscribe to Vegan Outreach's weekly eNewsletter and my own Vegan.com blog.

- Eat right and take the supplements you need to guarantee optimal health.

I've discovered that the more vegans learn about farmed animal issues, the more devoted they become to compassionate eating. Although they're hard to watch, factory farming videos like those available at MercyForAnimals.org will undoubtedly increase your commitment to be vegan. And there's nothing like connecting with the animals at a farmed animal sanctuary to further embrace a vegan lifestyle. People *go* vegan for any number of reasons, but they often *stay* vegan for the animals.

And remember: always celebrate your victories. You've just finished reading all my advice on how to go vegan. Take a few minutes to reflect on how much you've learned, and how much further you've progressed down the vegan path. I hope you've had a good time learning this material, and that it has set you up for a lifetime of healthy and satisfying vegan living.

Part III

Activism

"I have wasted my life playing video games.
Luckily, I have two extra lives."

—kNeil

Chapter **27**

Basic Activism & Outreach

If there's one thing I wish I could change about the vegetarian community, a single fact that frustrates and saddens me beyond belief, it's that most vegetarians view their personal diets as their sole form of animal advocacy. I doubt if one vegetarian in ten makes an unwavering effort to inform others about dietary issues.

There are doubtless many reasons why vegetarians rarely engage in outreach. They may not know where to begin. They may not know other activists with whom they might collaborate. Or they may fear that doing this work would brand them as zealots. But I think there is one reason above all else why so few vegetarians take up activism, and that is: the typical vegetarian has *no idea* how much animal suffering just a little activism can prevent. Not the slightest idea.

The fact is that even miniscule investments of time can produce massive results. How little time and how massive a result? Imagine this: it's probable that by investing just thirty minutes doing simple outreach, you'll keep as many animals out of factory farms and slaughterhouses as you would by following a totally vegan diet for the rest of your life.

I hope this assertion has you saying "where do I sign up?" That's easy: just visit VeganOutreach.org and join their Adopt-a-College program. This program enables you to protect huge numbers of animals for every hour that you participate.

The genius of the Adopt-a-College program lies in its ability to take advantage of the fact that most Westerners were raised with a profound disconnect. Most of us were taught from childhood to love animals and to be kind to them, yet nearly of all of us were brought up on a diet rich in animal products. It's tragic that most Americans make it all the way through high school without being exposed to information about factory farms and slaughterhouses. Yet this horrible situation does create an exciting possibility: college campuses offer tremendous opportunities for outreach. There, you've got thousands of young people congregated in one place, most of whom are on their own for the first time in their lives. Many of these students are remarkably receptive to learning about animal agriculture and re-evaluating their food choices. But for this to happen, somebody needs to distribute relevant information.

That's where you come in. As an Adopt-a-College volunteer, you visit your local college campus and pass out free booklets from Vegan Outreach. At a busy campus, it's easy to pass out a couple hundred booklets an hour. That's 200 people, for each hour invested, who would not receive this information if it were not for you. The results of this outreach effort are inspiring—astonishing even. Rarely does a day go by without reports coming in to Vegan Outreach from people who've received a booklet and decided to go vegan.

The beautiful thing about Adopt-a-College is that it requires no training, and can accommodate a commitment ranging from minimal to gigantic. My friend Joe Espinosa got involved with the program when it launched in 2003, and today he's passed out more than 150,000 pamphlets. Another activist friend, Stewart Solomon, regularly passes out more than 20,000 pamphlets each semester—he finds time to do this despite being both a parent and a full-time teacher. And all across the United States, small local teams of activists regularly hit festivals and concerts, often distributing thousands of pamphlets at a single event.

People like these are heroes to me. They deserve to regarded as "animal millionaires," in that each of these people has spared millions and millions of animals the ordeal of the factory farm and slaughterhouse.

Sharing

Nearly every semester, the Adopt-a-College campaign sets a new distribution record. An astounding 491,000 booklets were handed out during the spring 2008 semester. As somebody who dreams of a vegan world, and the day when the last remaining slaughterhouse is shuttered, I have put many hours into thinking about why the Adopt-a-College campaign enjoys such remarkable success. I've come to believe that much of this program's power rests upon a single principle: the effectiveness of sharing instead of creating.

As an Adopt-a-College volunteer, there's no need to participate in researching, writing, designing, or printing the pamphlets you hand out. Your sole responsibility is at once the simplest and most vital part of the process—distributing these pamphlets to as many people as possible.

Put another way, just four people are responsible for creating Vegan Outreach's literature, yet hundreds of people volunteer to hand out these pamphlets. And whether we're considering the Adopt-a-College program or we're looking at other highly successful activist efforts, the same pattern constantly appears: few creators and many, many sharers.

The lesson that Adopt-a-College teaches us is that the most valuable people in the vegetarian movement aren't the creators, but the sharers. The cardinal sin of animal advocacy is to duplicate effort, since this means time is being wasted creating that could instead be spent sharing. Yet, sadly, this duplication happens all the time.

One obvious area of duplicated effort concerns vegan blogs. There are currently well over a hundred different blogs devoted to vegan cooking. While many of these are excellent, you've got to wonder: how many vegan cooking blogs can one person actually read? Does a hundred different vegan cooking blogs, with most read by just a handful of people, best serve the animals' interests? Wouldn't it be better if there were only five outstanding vegan cooking blogs in existence, with the other 95 bloggers shifting their energies towards sharing—rather than creating—vegan information?

So when you feel the urge to create something new in order to promote vegetarianism, the wisest response is generally to strangle that impulse in its crib. Opportunities for sharing are everywhere, and new opportunities constantly emerge.

Now I'm acutely conscious of the fact that here I am admonishing people not to create—in the pages of a book that I myself have created. Adding to my sins is that I'm also a blogger. But since I publish Vegan.com, which I think offers something unique to the Internet, I hope I can be excused and that my advice does not come off as hypocritical. In any event, I have to say that the books and blog entries I write are no longer the part of my work that interests me most.

My main passion is studying different forms of veggie activism, and trying to inspire people to participate in the most effective efforts. Specifically, this whole notion of sharing rather than creating is something I find endlessly interesting. As a result, even though I still create materials for the vegan community, I do this within a framework I hope others will follow.

This framework is easily summarized: *create only as a last resort.* I believe there are only two occasions when creation is more effective than putting that same time and energy into sharing. First, is when what you're creating is fundamentally new and different—when the core quality of what you're creating just hasn't been captured by anyone else in the veggie movement. And second, it can make sense to duplicate efforts if you've identified a resource that already exists, but that you're somehow capable of improving on by leaps and bounds.

Vegan Outreach co-founder Matt Ball regularly emphasizes to aspiring activists that you don't need to start a group or organize anything to make a real difference. Happily, there's no shortage of great vegan-oriented materials and projects. But there is a terrible scarcity of vegans who are willing to participate in basic outreach efforts.

Admittedly, the prospect of leafletting by yourself may seem intimidating. You may therefore find it worthwhile to become acquainted with other activists, who you might team up with for leafletting efforts. Hundreds of cities and towns have regular vegan dinner gatherings, and Meetup.com is a great place to find these events. Likewise, it can be worthwhile to attend one of the many large vegetarian or animal rights conferences that takes place each year, as these events offer unsurpassed opportunities for networking.

However you choose to do it, I urge you to just grit your teeth and get out there. Order a box of brochures from VeganOutreach.org, circle a date on your calendar, and then follow through on your commitment to leaflet on that day. Nothing feels better than coming home after a couple of hours spent leafletting, knowing that you've just gotten dozens of people to think about eating more compassionately.

Leafletting is just one way to share vegan information. Advertising is another exciting approach.

Advertising

The vegan movement may never be able to buy advertising on the scale that McDonald's does. Fortunately, there are all sorts of effective advertising opportunities available to activists that come at little or no cost.

Email Signatures

When you think of advertising, you may envision large corporate firms occupying prestigious office towers, designing million-dollar ads for the Super Bowl.

Yet there is a wonderful advertising opportunity available that doesn't even cost a nickel, and is ideally suited to vegetarian advocacy. Just about every free email service allows you to create a custom signature for the emails you send out. And if you use a dedicated email client, such as Thunderbird or Outlook, you can likewise set up a signature there a well. From that moment forward, every email you send will have your own personal vegetarian advocacy message attached to the bottom.

Why let this free opportunity go to waste? My only advice is to keep your blurb short, and link to a website that offers more information. Some links you may wish to include are your favorite vegan blog, hand-picked online recipes, and Vegan Outreach's website. It makes sense to offer two or more links in your signature: for instance, one for general vegan information and another for food and recipes.

Bumper Stickers

After email signatures, the cheapest advertising campaign I know of costs only a dollar or two, and will be seen by thousands of people during its lifetime. It is the humble bumper sticker. I think it's best to promote your favorite vegan website rather than have a bumper sticker featuring some lame "don't eat the animals" slogan. That way, your bumper sticker provides a comprehensive source of information to anyone who's interested. The best vegan websites offer snazzy bumper stickers—you can easily find these at any big veggie festival or animal rights conference.

One final piece of advice where bumper stickers are concerned: choose your favorite sticker and stop at one per car. Multiple stickers mean multiple messages, whereas a single clear message is easier for people to absorb and act on. If there's one point that vegan activists need to be constantly reminded of, it's to keep their message simple, well-chosen, and memorable: brevity is key.

Television and Billboards

Vegan Outreach has shown that handing out literature where young people congregate can deliver enormous results when it comes to protecting animals. Now imagine taking this approach a step further and going straight into people's living rooms to distribute this information. Amazingly, this task can be accomplished without risking arrest for breaking and entering: all you need to do is donate money to purchase television ads.

At least two groups, Mercy For Animals and Compassion Over Killing, regularly create short, punchy, youth-oriented television ads that promote vegan diets. Many cable companies sell regional advertising slots on MTV and other networks that cater to young people. It can be surprisingly cheap—just a few cents per viewer—to purchase these ads. So, for activists with more money than time, or anyone who wouldn't feel comfortable handing out leaflets, the purchase of these ads can expose thousands of people to a vegan message at a low cost.

Money spent on television advertising slots can go a long way, since the ads themselves have already been written, produced, and paid for. Nonprofits often allow donors to earmark their contribution specifically to purchasing blocks of advertising time from cable companies.

In addition to television, there are other forms of advertising worth considering. Some animal protection groups, such as Mercy For Animals, have created billboards and bus advertisements. Here again, for a relatively small donation, you can purchase advertising space that will expose thousands of people to a vegan message.

Beyond the Basics

Even a brand new vegetarian can implement any of the ideas presented in this chapter. But nothing here is exclusively for beginners—even long-term and highly accomplished activists regularly participate in much of the work I've described. For instance, Paul Shapiro, who heads up the factory farming campaign for the Humane Society of the United States, will still spend a Saturday afternoon passing out leaflets. And nearly all experienced activists I've encountered have a well-chosen bumper sticker affixed to their cars, plus they also include some sort of vegetarian advocacy message in their email signatures.

There are of course other sorts of activism that have much higher barriers to entry—techniques that require expertise and abilities that are beyond the reach of novice activists. Appendix A provides an introduction to some of the possibilities for advanced animal protection work. But there's no need to take up specialized activism: you can prevent enormous amounts of animal suffering by doing only the basic techniques described in this chapter.

Perhaps the animals' greatest hope is the fact that anyone who cares enough to act, and who contributes either time or money towards simple outreach efforts, can spare millions upon millions of animals from a lifetime of suffering. A vegan world will only become possible if the majority of vegans wake up to the enormous power they possess.

Appendices

Appendix A: Advanced Activism

Given sufficient commitment, it's possible for one person to keep millions and millions of animals out of the slaughterhouse by following the advice offered in the final chapter of this book. That said, some people will want to take on more complex and demanding activist opportunities. So this appendix is intended to offer guidance to activists who are seeking out tougher challenges and even bigger rewards.

But please know that unless you feel a calling to become deeply involved in animal protection work, there's no need to follow any of the advice presented here. You can accomplish enormous good for the animals without going beyond any of the advice I offered in this book's final chapter.

With that caveat out of the way, my advice for advanced activism boils down to three overarching tasks. First, you will need to become an expert in topics related to vegetarianism and animal protection. Second, you must identify people who carry great influence on how others eat. And third, you'll then develop relationships with these people, so that they'll depend on you to keep them informed about vegan topics.

Developing Expertise

The process of developing expertise begins by reading heavily. And here, you'll encounter your first hazard, since many of the books in the vegetarian literature are loaded with misinformation. To help you clear that initial obstacle, I've hand-picked several of the most accurate titles for this book's recommended reading section (see Appendix B).

The reading you do shouldn't be limited to books; blogs are another great place to stay informed about vegan-oriented news. I update the Vegan.com blog throughout the week, and you can discover numerous other blogs and online sources that regularly feature important information.

Becoming widely read in the veggie literature is the easy part of developing your expertise. The harder part involves learning how to evaluate competing claims, and to assess the accuracy of a book, scientific report, or article. Difficult as it is to develop, this ability is absolutely necessary for anyone who aspires to be considered an expert in a given field. There's no reason to become an expert in order to do basic activism like adopting a college—your job is merely to share quality information, and you can rely on the fine people at Vegan Outreach to make sure this information is carefully researched and overwhelmingly accurate. But once you seek expert status, the burden of analyzing the accuracy of the information you read falls on your shoulders. Having the ability to discriminate between reliable and unreliable information is key, since when you pass along information that turns out to be false, you lose credibility—and, as an expert, your credibility is all you have.

So it's critical that you develop your analytical skills. Here, people with a background in science or law have a big head start. Success in these fields demands cultivating a skeptical disposition, and knowing how to probe a given claim for weaknesses.

One way or another, whether through professional training

or through cultivating your own analytical skills, every expert needs a reliable B.S. detector. The key to seeing through bad information is to learn how to ask questions that reveal a claim's credibility.

The first question to ask is, "who is making this claim and why should I trust them?" A fact reported by *The New York Times* may be incorrect, but it's nevertheless far more likely to be true than something published by a small-town newspaper with extreme political views.

Some information sources are far more reliable than even the best newspapers. If you've found a study published by the United Nations or *The New England Journal of Medicine*, you've got a great source. Better still is a review article, published by a prestigious journal, that references a hundred reputable studies that have all reported the same thing. By contrast, a blog entry claiming that milk is poison, but which does not offer a citation for this claim, is not a reputable source.

Finally, on even minor points, you must always ask: does the claim itself seem reasonable? Lacking solid documentation, you've got to ask if a given piece of information passes the sniff test. If an item doesn't seem like it could be true, and there's no strong evidence supporting it, you're best off assuming it's false.

Identifying and Befriending Opinion Leaders

Once you've developed your expertise, how do you put it to use?

In a perfect world, you could snap your fingers and gain a huge following of people who would hang on your every word. But attracting a large and faithful audience is a daunting task, whereas gaining the attention of one person with great influence is comparatively easy. People with great influence are called opinion leaders—just one opinion leader can inspire large numbers of people to rethink their opinions and behavior. Whenever an opinion leader takes an interest in your work, the gains are potentially massive. Let me tell a couple quick stories to illustrate this point. As you'll see, there are many kinds of opinion leaders and many ways to get their attention.

The Blogger

The first story I'll share involves a connection I personally formed with an opinion leader. My blog at Vegan.com is currently small potatoes; if I post something there only a few thousand people will see it. But every once in a while I'll encounter a story that I think deserves to be seen by millions. This will of course never happen if all I do is post the story to Vegan.com.

Happily, I've gradually gained the attention of a contributor to one of the top blogs on the web, BoingBoing.net, which gets millions of visitors each day. Mark Frauenfelder is not a vegan, but I love the stories he posts, and over time I've developed a precise feel for the topics that grab his interest.

Every once in a while, a pro-vegan or anti-meat story comes along that has a compelling hook, one that I know would interest Mark. On those occasions, I'll write up the story for Vegan.com, and then follow up this post with a very brief email to Mark. Because I follow Mark's work closely, I'm able to reliably anticipate the sorts of stories that capture his interest. As a consequence, most of the times I send Mark a story he decides to run it.

There are three keys to my successful relationship with Mark. The first key is that I am an expert in a subject that is of interest to him. The second key is that I pay attention to Mark's work, so that I know the sorts of things that he finds most interesting. And the third key is the most important of all: the restraint I bring to our relationship.

Mark is a busy guy, and as one of the world's most influential bloggers he's got plenty of people competing for his attention. So I have to exercise the utmost restraint when it comes to contacting him. Every day, I see stories that *might* interest Mark. But might is nowhere near good enough. Email is an interruption-based form of communication, and if you interrupt somebody the payback to them better be worthwhile. If not, your relationship erodes with each new interruption, and your recipient will quickly reach the point where he'll ignore all of your emails.

So I only email Mark on the rarest of occasions, maybe a half-dozen times each year, and only when I've found a story I'm certain will interest him. Because of the restraint I show when it comes to contacting Mark, he knows that each of the very rare emails he receives from me contains something of genuine interest.

And that, in a nutshell, is how you turn yourself into an opinion leader's trusted source. That person might be a successful blogger, a business leader, or a reporter—it doesn't matter; the steps to gaining and holding an opinion leader's attention are the same.

The Business Leader

In 2001, lauren[1] Ornelas was working with a nonprofit that was trying to convince Whole Foods Market to stop selling duck meat sourced from factory farms. Initial overtures to the company produced discouraging results, but at a company shareholder meeting Ornelas finally succeeded at establishing a line of communication to the CEO, John Mackey.

Their dialog began with Ornelas questioning whether Whole Foods' animal welfare standards were meaningful, and she challenged Mackey to learn more about the issues. Mackey was impressed by Ornelas' passion for animal protection, so he took the initiative to read a number of books related to factory farming and veganism.

After completing this reading, Mackey switched to a near-vegan diet. He then embarked on a series of initiatives that raised the animal welfare standards at Whole Foods Market substan-

---

[1]Not a typo: lauren doesn't capitalize her first name.

tially above those of any competing supermarket chain. Mackey describes Ornelas as the spark that helped him to go vegan and make animal welfare issues a personal concern.

Just as we saw regarding my interactions with Mark Frauenfelder, Ornelas' story shows what opening a dialog with the right person can accomplish. By being informed, respectful, and offering a concisely stated message that relates to your recipient's personal interests, it's possible to get highly influential people to do things that dramatically advance the vegan cause.

Social Networking

I'm going to finish this appendix by briefly covering the activism topic that currently interests me most: Internet-based social networking. This is a subject that's so new, and changing so rapidly, that I can only offer a few specific pieces of advice. But the appeal is undeniable. Social networking websites have the ability to put you in communication with countless people who share your interests, in effect handing you the tools to become a virtual opinion leader.

I won't pretend to understand all the ways these sites can be used for the sake of protecting animals, but there are several simple and obvious things that anyone can do. The first is to put veggie-oriented information on your MySpace and Facebook pages. This information can include books you recommend, photos that are of interest, relevant websites, and finally some quotes or statistics about the subject.

Always strive to distill your points to their essence. On your main MySpace page, it's better to put up two great photos than twenty, and five worthwhile books and websites rather than fifty. There's probably nothing more ineffective than a page that takes five minutes to load because it's overrun with photos, random images, and video. Sadly, perhaps half the MySpace users I've encountered who are committed to activism choke off the effectiveness of their page by crowding it, willy-nilly, with too many images and too much information. Discipline and restraint carry the day when creating an effective vegan-oriented social networking profile.

So, your first priority is to make sure your personal social networking pages concisely present the most relevant vegetarian-oriented information. With that accomplished, you can use status updates to announce news or recipes that you find of interest. Here again, restraint pays off—update your Facebook status too often and people will stop paying attention to you.

Finally, you can use social networking news and resource sites like Digg, Yahoo Buzz, and StumbleUpon to highlight stories you want people in your circle to know about. Using these news-oriented sites effectively can be a challenge, since each of these sites has its own special tricks for gaining influence within its community. But one overarching strategy delivers big payoffs on all these websites: you've got to find and add friends who share your interests so that you can co-promote one anothers' most interesting posts.

Using social networking tools to gain influence is hard work. The websites are often complex and evolving, and so there are few clearly-defined ways for a newcomer to gain influence. Yet by frequenting these online communities and paying attention to what its most influential members do, it's possible to glimpse strategies that will enable you to reach large numbers of people.

It's fun to play around with social networking sites to look for ways your activism can hit a home run. But until you get your big break, it's wise to spend most of your time using the tried-and-true activist techniques covered in this book's final chapter.

Appendix B: Books, Websites, & Nonprofits

Books:

Marcus, Erik. *Meat Market*
Regan, Tom. *Empty Cages*
Shirky, Clay. *Here Comes Everybody*
Singer, Peter. *Animal Liberation*

Websites:

Barnivore.com
FatFreeVegan.com
Meetup.com
RobinRobertson.com
Vegan.com
VeganEatingOut.com

Nonprofits:

Compassion Over Killing (COK.net)
Compassionate Action for Animals (CA4A.org)
Mercy For Animals (MercyForAnimals.org)
Vegan Outreach (VeganOutreach.org)

Appendix C: Vegan-Friendly Beers

Here's a handy list of 25 popular vegan beers and breweries.

- Anchor Steam and all Anchor beers

- Anderson Valley Brewing Company

- Budweiser & Bud Light (Anheuser-Busch sponsors rodeos)

- Chimay

- Coors

- Corona

- Flying Dog Brewery

- Full Sail Brewing Co.

- Geary Brewing Company

- Harpoon Brewery

- Heineken (but it tastes like piss)

- Lagunitas (everything but Olde GnarlyWine is vegan)

- Lost Coast Brewery

- Magic Hat Brewing Company

- McMenamins (unless milk or honey is in the beer's name)

- Miller Genuine Draft and Miller Lite

- North Coast Brewing Company

- Pabst Blue Ribbon

- Pyramid Breweries

- Redhook Ale Brewery

- Rolling Rock (Anheuser-Busch sponsors rodeos)

- Sam Adams (except Cherry Wheat and Honey Porter)

- Sierra Nevada Brewing Company

- Smuttynose Brewing Company

- Unibroue Inc.

For a complete and constantly-updated directory of all vegan-friendly beers and wines, visit Barnivore.com.

Appendix D: Cashew Cheese

People have been asking for my cashew cheese recipe ever since I mentioned it in *Vegan: The New Ethics of Eating.* Cashew cheese is a perfect pizza topping, and it's also great on grilled cheese sandwiches. Eating it with sprouts on a bagel may also make you happy.

Ingredients

1 cup raw unsalted cashews
2 Tablespoons raw tahini
$\frac{1}{4}$ **of an average-sized chopped red bell pepper**
1 Tablespoon tamari
1 Tablespoon olive oil
1 Tablespoon nutritional yeast

Directions

Put all above ingredients in food processor and process with blade until completely smooth. In a pinch, you can use a blender to do this, but chances are you'll need to dilute the mixture with water to attain proper smoothness.

Index

Vegan.com

Erik Marcus publishes Vegan.com, a leading source of information, news, and recipes for the animal protection community.

1553076